Challenges

of

Challenging Behaviour

A CARER'S HAND BOOK
A REFERENCE BOOK FOR THE STUDENT OF CHALLENGING BEHAVIOUR,
THE "SPECIAL EDUCATION NEEDS COORDINATOR" (SENCO).
A SUPPORT HANDBOOK FOR CARERS, PARENTS, SOCIAL WORKERS, TEACHERS
NURSERY NURSES AND CHILDMINDERS

BY: IBRAHIM NELSON KAGGWA

ACKNOWLEDGEMENTS

Special appreciation to:
My Publicists;
Gwen and David Morrison
Of
"PUBLISH NATION"
For making the publication of this book possible.

Special appreciation to:
Nasreen Begum-Kaggwa (A very special person in all)
Ayesha B-K (Challenging me to rewrite and re-start whenever she switched off my computer)
Aminah B-K (For various text contributions and the psychedelic cover design)
Mariam B-K (For the technical input for cover design)

-   Sheffield Rygate Children's Centre
-   Sheffield Children's Hospital
-   UK KIDZ Colleagues
The specialists whose many training sessions I have attended and for what they do for many children

To

My Parents the best carers ever

CONTENTS

INTRODUCTION:

This book is a study, a course; a reference book; focussed on particular and generally addressing how to care for those with "challenging behaviour". Challenging behaviour results from various circumstances; it is triggered. Start from the notion that everything has a cause. The book is the result of some personal experience, professional training, and understanding of caring for children or individuals that exhibit challenging behaviour. Therefore, I write it in the first-person context. It is about me and you; how I see things which you may experience but encounter differently. The book helps any prospective carer who could be a student learning to care, a parent, SENCO, teacher, or a professional carer. The book is written in a British environment and context.

Challenging behaviour is incredibly complex and challenging. Challenging behaviour is often looked at as a disability. It is deplorable that disability continues to be used by many in society to determine the circumstance and future of individuals: I believe that a child's disability should not define their future. Challenging behaviour in my view ranges from the mundane to the extreme: the child refusing food, failing to learn to talk, the autistic child, the one who is dyslexic, the one with Asperger's syndrome, the one who has "Impulse and addiction control disorder" (IACD), eating disorders such as anorexia nervosa, psychotic disorders, e.g. schizophrenia, delusion, and others. This book is for the carer and parent needing to learn good practice for day-to-day survival. It is a book to help us survive the moment, not a medical solution. It is to help us understand the child or individual we are caring for and how we can survive with their needs.

The child with Crohn's is the one who works so hard so fast to ensure the onset of Crohn's pains do not catch her in the middle of her work. People think she works at supersonic speed, yet she is rushing against time, against her different ability. The child who has "Avoidant Restrictive Food Intake Disorder" (ARFID) always smells the food from a distance and is one that survives on milk in the main; she refuses most solid food, just wants to eat fish and chicken popcorn; yet she is the one always ready to share her food (!!!!), very kind to others but not to herself. Be kind to get rid of the food. The autistic child is the one able to draw psychedelic pictures that dazzle. Those that know nothing about art think she's done something wrong! Yet she exhibits a different ability.

Challenging behaviour is always exhibited in different degrees: challenging behaviour may not be a disability but a different ability: the autistic child is more observant than the rest of the family, she has a stronger sense of smell than the rest of her peers, she will tell the time for things to happen without looking at a clock or a watch, she has that intuition that does not naturally come to others: she can draw exact replicas of things or scenes as observed. She is more analytical and amazes many in her design and artistic work. She exhibits a sensitivity of love and care that is exceptional. Challenging behaviour is exceptional: the complexity for society and professionals is that individuals with challenging behaviour are challenging society, challenging you and me. That is the challenge to you and all. Individuals with challenging behaviour are challenging the deficiencies in carers. It is a different ability: how we respond to that different ability is keenly observed and analysed by the child/individual with challenging behaviour. Those with challenging conditions wonder why we the carers, parents, and professionals panic when they have onsets of their conditions or attacks, they wonder why we are not positive when they resist, and wonder why we do not plan, to forewarn them of things that will change their routine.

The abilities of the child or individual exhibiting challenging behaviour are a different ability, not a disability. Disability is only in the mind of the observer, whereas the individual with challenging behaviour is able in more ways than one. Whilst we put much effort in containing and think we are observing them, they are observing us and analysing how we treat them, how we are with them, and our attitudes are towards them. This book is focussing on enabling the carer to be positive and work with the child or individual with dignity and a positive attitude. Challenging behaviour is not necessarily mental illness; there are many conditions that trigger challenges in behaviours of individuals. The most constructive way for a carer or parent to deal with challenging behaviour is to accept the challenge and respond in a positive and caring manner.

IS IT A CHALLENGING STORY?

When confronted with a situation, you find that you need to address it. A carer is confronted with an individual with a need; thereby the situation demands action, a response to the challenge posed. A child behaving in a way that is unusual, unexpected, and challenging what we would call norms of life, may be exhibiting signs of challenging behaviour. Challenging behaviour carers are steered by behavioural professionals to focus so much on "disorder and disability". In this book it is preferred to focus on challenges posed to the carer by the "challenging behaviour". The challenge is a need expressed by the individual or child; the child or individual wants something done, given to, or dealt with for them. This book is to support, so that we should be able to meet needs whilst ensuring we do not get overwhelmed in the process of providing care. Anyone can exhibit challenging behaviour depending on circumstances. A distraught and bereaved individual could easily fit the characterisation of challenging behaviour. Children like stories especially if they are funny, but also if they are perplexing and exciting: the following little story is told so we draw positive images out of would-be "disorders".

Once upon a war; a warlord was injured in a battle. He lost an eye and a leg. He was a ruthless man who did not take kindly to any type of negative criticism. But he was the head of a large tribe and in the stately home he occupied as residence, where there were many portraits of the former preceding leaders of his tribe. One day as he gazed around at these portraits he got an idea that his portrait be painted beautifully and hung up there on the wall while he was still ruler.

He commanded that all painters from near and far be called so he could commission a painter for his portrait: when all painters were gathered interviews were done and all the painters but one came up with all manner of excuses why they could not draw the portrait. The reality was they were scared to do a realistic portrait due to his disabilities. (Sadly many people in this modern world think that those of us with one type or other, visible or invisible disability, would be offended if the disability is pointed out. The challenge is if our needs are not pointed out how then can the carer care meeting those needs in a targeted way?) The painter who stood up got commissioned and started working, producing a very beautiful portrait: it was of the leader holding an arrow and bow, one eye open of course, and was astride a horse, such that the amputated leg was not showing. Oh dear! The leader was pleased, but challenged the painter that: "Don't hide my disability of my amputated leg; let future generations see that even in that condition my people accepted me as their leader; let future youths with disabilities be inspired that they can lead, and excel; let future generations and those present today learn not to bully anyone or demean anyone because of visible or invisible disabilities."

This book shows the challenges of challenging behaviour, and uses various examples and in particular those faced in childcare.

The book is to support the carer to do what is needed for the child or adult individual who shows challenging behaviour.

CHAPTER 1

The challenge posed by the meaning of challenging behaviour

This is the simple explanation of what is meant by the terms "behaviour that challenges" and "positive behaviour".

a) Behaviour that challenges:

There is a common trait among professionals in health and care to term or name every unusual condition a "disorder". Why they do this is an academic discussion. In behaviour studies, there is a tendency to label individuals who behave differently as having "challenging behaviour". This is purely because of the observer; "you" view them differently; "you" are challenged by their ways, and then you blame them for how they are instead of accepting them and respecting them and treating them with the dignity they so much deserve. Through the experience of how a child or an adult acts, we should understand that: challenging behaviour is considered so if it poses those around to question why it is happening: for instance: why does this child continue to wet the bed at the age of ten? Has this child got a weak bladder or is s/he oblivious to the need to go to the toilet or is it something that needs investigating? Why does the toddler always cry and cover her ears with her hands whenever the washing machine or vacuum cleaner is turned on? Has this child got sensory issues? Behaviour is considered challenging if it is also a risk or harmful to the individual or to others and leads the sufferer and those around them to have a poor quality of life. It serves to show that the individual and the environment they are in are not working in tandem.

b) Positive behaviour:

Positive behaviour is that which ensures that the child's needs or an individual's needs are met; it involves both words and actions. It ensures the well-being and dignity of the individual and others around that individual. To secure positive before therefore demands from the parent, the SENCO, and the carer an affirmative attitude, to reassure and offer dignity to the child or individual exhibiting behaviour that challenges us. The positive behaviour enables us to realise full potential in ourselves and for the child or individual we are caring for.

A carer, parent, or teacher should use the following information to identify examples of verbal, non-verbal, and physical behaviour that could be perceived as challenging.

a) Verbal behaviour:

There is a clear comprehension according to the professional definition: verbal behaviour is challenging if the individual is; acting contrary to the expected norm; shouting, arguing, abusive, or offending in use of inappropriate language in their communication; the individual may also be threatening verbally, calling names, or using words and terms that are inappropriate such as discriminative sexist or racist terms.

b) Non-verbal behaviour:

To understand non-verbal behaviour we need knowledge: this book simply teaches you that perceived non-verbal behaviours can include unpleasantness of rude looks and deliberate negative facial expressions. Non-verbal behaviour can also be silence in a deliberate form. It can be rudely walking away when being spoken to. Deliberately clenching of fists and waving of, e.g. the index finger into people's faces. Invading space by standing in a threatening manner into another person's personal space. In some instances non-verbal behaviour can just result into screaming, putting on an aggressive posture, or pointing into another person's face.

c) Physical behaviour:

The subcategories of challenging physical behaviour are four, namely: Self-harm, Stereotypical, Direct aggression, Non-person direct.

- Self-harm challenging physical behaviour is mammoth and may include overeating or under-eating food. It can also be evidenced in eating or chewing on non-food items, including objects or substances that may be poison. Individuals in this condition can gouge or poke their own eyes, self-harm; they grind teeth, bang their heads against walls, pulling their hair out, or in instances deliberately burn themselves.

- Stereotyped challenging behaviour can include the individual making repetitive movements, rocking from side to side or forward to back, or pacing about aimlessly, and making repetitive speech.

- Directly aggressive will evidence such behaviour as spitting, pulling of hair, nail biting, biting self or others, intimidation, and hitting or punching when anyone gets into close space. Children will do poking or scratching and pinch other children. Kicking and throwing objects without considering danger. This behaviour can also be seen where an individual corners others.

- The non-person directed subcategory of challenging physical behaviour is usually seen in the individual's lack of awareness; they may have no sense of danger or have poor judgement of anticipation. They can even steal, behave sexually inappropriately, be withdrawn, and in many cases be suffering from incontinence.

Behaviour may potentially impact the individual's own and others' feelings and attitudes in the short term and long term.

To understand and describe how the behaviour may potentially impact the individual's own and others' feelings and attitudes in the short and long term is to deal with hypothetical questions which are in the care industry real. It is important to emphasise here that the impact and effects of behaviour that challenges on others may be vast and the care worker must have a concept of time, circumstances, and situation, so that the care worker/provider clearly takes measures of self-protection, taking care of themselves whilst carrying out the role of care not just to be safe, but also avoid burning out from exhaustion or exacerbation: yet the care worker must be aware of the result of any care actions taken for the individual that suffers behaviour that challenges, since there are the short-term and long term impacts or effects on that individual: the situation that arises from short-, medium-, or long-term effects and impact of behaviour that challenges and who it affects can be described more clearly as follows: to deal with this particular issue we may use two strands:

- The individual or sufferer of behaviour that challenges

- The "others" who relate or come in contact with the individual who exhibits behaviour that challenges

STRAND 1. Impact on Individual/Sufferer.

- In the short term:

The challenging behaviour impacts on the individual or the sufferer: the sufferer could, if they are a nursery child, be put on time-out, and if they were for instance a youth offender, could have such privileges as access to phone or sports withheld.

When impacted in that way,

- In the long term:

The individual may become anxious and this may culminate in becoming depressed. A child that has a learning disability may not learn anything from the time-out, and then shows even more excessive challenging behaviour. In that situation the withdrawal of privileges would not work, but a calming-down method may help. It must be clear that no action is taken to be mistaken as reward.

- In the short term:

There may occur impacts or effects that are physical such as injury. The individual may have self-harmed or came into collision with objects due to their challenging behaviour. There then occurs an immediate action to provide emergency care to stop, e.g. bleeding or further self-injury and/or harm.

- In the long term:

Individuals with behaviour that challenges have been known to feel disrespect and humiliation because they have been put under restraint due to the way they behaved. It is in many cases evident that since the restraint is not desirable, the individual may become upset, anxious, and depressed in the long term. For instance if protective gloves were put on the hands of one who is scratching themselves, they may feel humiliated, that it is undesirable for their hands to be restrained.

- In the short term:

The individual that has behaviour that challenges may get short-term impact through positive use of rewards from carers. When reward is given, the impact may be that good behaviour is achieved and relief is gotten away from behaviour that challenges.

- In the long term:

Individuals or sufferers of challenging behaviour can in the long term resort to attempts of caring for themselves or finding survival techniques which may be dangerous; for example they can resort to drug abuse, overdosing, or get relief from alcohol. These things are done by the individual in an attempt to self-manage, self-enable, yet wrongly; to respond to any privilege withheld, or to counter restraint they may be subjected to.

- In the short term:

When behaviour that challenges is being managed, the individual may be placed into voluntary segregation or isolation: this sort of situation arises where the individual requests that they be isolated as they feel sorry for their actions of challenging behaviour. The short-term impact is their feeling of being singled out or isolation from others.

- In the long term:

When isolated and without carer support the individual may be taken advantage of by unscrupulous people, becoming the subject of abuse especially if they are children: isolation comes about from the individual who, when isolated, can resort to becoming avoidant, reluctant, and refusing to use services of care which are needed. This can cause vulnerability and is likely to result in deterioration of the individual's overall health and well-being condition.

STRAND 2. Impact on others:

In the short term:

"Others" who come face to face with the "individual" with behaviour that challenges may get the impact of being "shocked" or very surprised and the surprise may be distressing or scary. These "others" may be the carer themselves. And where a carer becomes shocked there is need for commanding skills that have been learned to manage that situation.

In the long term:

The others that encounter with behaviour that challenges could themselves fail to share experiences of shock and internalise trauma, which then makes them isolated. The life of the carer can be overwhelmed, the carer's tasks and role overtake the life of the carer, and the carer cannot manage and begins to live a poor quality of life. The effects of such overwhelming can make carers not meet their personal responsibilities. It is important a carer draws from professional support from colleagues or professional services if they are caring for a family member.

In the short term:

Impact and effects on a carer who finds themselves with a family member that has behaviour that challenges may suffer embarrassment. For example a child with autism may wave their hands and hit passers-by who are unaware of the special need: the parent may be placed in an embarrassing situation of having to apologise and explain. Or in an instance where a family member that suffers from Crohn's disease and is desperately seeking a toilet, embarrassment could occur. Whilst the short-term impact is embarrassment, the sufferer and the carer are impacted long-term.

In the long term:

Impact or effects on others; e.g. for myself as a family carer with children that have special needs, I have found myself angry and resentful of the situation I find myself in. This happens when I cannot do what I want to do because of the needs of the children; e.g. I may want to eat a burger takeaway, but have to consider how it will affect my child that has Crohn's. There is therefore long-term impact seen in the disruption of planning what to buy, what to cook, and what to eat. The caring role does make an impact on others, not just the carer, but even when planning a meal that involves visitors we have to think twice.

In the short term:

Impact on "others" or carers may be subjected to physical injury; for example I am a trustee in a childcare provision, where I have seen children with behaviour that challenges use their teeth to bite, and the carer/teacher has to act fast to help the individual unlearn the habit of biting. The physical injury may demand immediate action. In adult care the injury to the "other(s)" may be even more severe than a child's bite, e.g. if challenging behaviour involves the individual who throws objects or even is physically strong and attacks.

In the long term:

Impact on carers could find themselves in worsening or deteriorating situations when their own well-being is affected; the self-esteem of a mother caring for a violent teenager can be of loss of self-esteem. A wife that cares for an alcoholic abusive husband can become negatively impacted. In some instance when the condition of the individual with behaviour that challenges persists the carer can feel inadequate, not doing the job correctly, resulting in self-blame.

In the short term:

Impact or effects on "others" who are carers or those that encounter or have to deal with individuals with behaviour that challenges may have to make firm decisions; these are referred to as assertive decisions professionally. This is done by others to ensure that there is a stop to the behaviour that challenges; e.g. if the individual is attacking others or the carer, restraint may take a medical method to subdue the individual in order to prevent danger or injury to self and others.

In the long term:

Impact or effects on others who work as staff in situations where there is behaviour that challenges can result into the loss of self-confidence, but also the loss of trust in those who exhibit such behaviour, or if the behaviour is exhibited by a colleague the others may be made to feel inferior, intimidated, or inadequate. It is also possible that such carers can then begin to overexert themselves and experience professional burnout.

In the short term:

The impact or effects on others could be a feeling of exacerbation or utter frustration: (a) that the behaviour that challenges is not going away, (b) that the behaviour that challenges was not stopped earlier. In these two instances it is difficult to call on hindsight as life is unpredictable. The carer can only treat the present condition. The past may have contributed, but present action, care, or treatment can help make the future better: care can make life liveable for family carers who deal with situations of behaviour that challenges. Frustrations experienced by carers or others that encounter behaviour that challenges need to be shared by them with their mentors, colleagues, and discussed in order to address the root cause of such frustrations.

In the long term:

The "others" or those who encounter or deal with individuals with behaviour that challenges may be impacted with long-term labelling. Some staff work in a particular way, e.g. where poor timekeeping is common an individual may be described as irresponsible, or where an individual makes light of serious situations, they can be labelled flippant. And where inflexibility is exhibited an individual can easily be described as difficult. It is essential, therefore, in care to always negotiate with others working in a team to arrive at policy and appropriate actions to avoid being put in a frustrating situation which may lead to being labelled when working in a situation of supporting those who have behaviour that challenges.

In summary this book is a course of study enabling me, the carer, to understand that it is important to always consider:

How behaviour that challenges may impact:

- The individual and others

- The feelings and attitudes of the individual and that of others

- In the environment/circumstances of community, in the short and long term

CHAPTER 2

The challenge of the reasons causing people to present challenging behaviour

BEHAVIOUR CAN BE INTERPRETED AS A FORM OF EXPRESSION:

Foremost the parent or carer and teacher must understand that any behaviour is in the perception of observers. It is the observer that sees, the seer that understands what is being exhibited. So when you are faced with challenging behaviour, it is you perceiving the challenge. You are being challenged; the parental skills you have, your carer skills, and your teacher skills are being challenged, tested, and demanded: how you respond to the need is your challenge.

Understanding "behaviour" helps us to interpret "it" as a form of expression: expression by individuals is a means by which they are understood and having needs met. Therefore where challenging behaviour is exhibited it simply is an expression. Without specialist understanding and empathy, the individual with challenging behaviour could be misunderstood, as their behaviour may not be the ordinary or it may be misinterpreted. In care work, professional training helps the variety of means by which individual expressions are interpreted and understood. Without specialist knowledge the life of individuals expressing themselves in challenging behaviour could fail to realise their full potential and having their needs met. This study has thus far enabled me to see that it is important to make a clear definition and description of behaviour being interpreted as a form of expression; e.g. a baby crying could be having a wet nappy or could be hungry: it is important that the mother or carer needs to interpret that expression of behaviour; and what the causes are.

It may not be what you immediately think, as behaviour may be a symptom of something else:

It is important to make a correct interpretation of behaviour. This is because that behaviour could be expressing an underlying symptom that needs addressing. Behaviour could be "a crying-out, a shouting-out" for help. A child going through domestic violence may in school express behaviour that challenges due to that experience. The child's frequent cause of particular is different from the basic behaviours that relate to common needs, e.g. basic needs such as water, sleep, warmth, or food; therefore the responses would be: if hungry, food is given; or if hot, coolant is provided. It is important to understand symptoms in work environments when providing care, so that expressions are understood in order to give appropriate responses to fulfil needs. Individuals with special needs could become increasingly agitated and this causes the onset of aggression when their expressed need is not met, e.g. a child wanting food may cry, and cry more as the hunger increases. Therefore, behaviour may be a symptom of something else.

Some examples of possible reasons for challenging behaviour:

There are many reasons for behaviour that challenges: examples of possible reasons for behaviour that challenges differ from situation to situation, and from one individual to another. The reasons include the following:

- Biological and physical: which determine "specific health conditions", maybe making the individual emotional, self-harm. It may be a genetic issue, e.g. a person that is violent or docile. It may be expressed in temperament. It can be sensory; where, e.g. a person has no sense of danger. It can also be failure to communicate feelings such as hunger or thirst needs. In cases of incontinence, there may be a failure by the sufferer to verbally express the need that they want to use the toilet, or fail physically to feel the urge or demand to use the toilet.

- Social: A child could refuse going to school, e.g. due to fear of being bullied. The fear of strangers may cause an individual to avoid crowds or just be antisocial. To be in the undesirable environment may cause stress and the resultant challenging behaviour; e.g. a child may feign illness or individuals may refuse to get out of an hour or car to avoid crowds. Darkness and/or lighting: people who suffer particular conditions such as hearing or visual and other physical conditions may be sensitive to the flashing or dimmed lighting of discos or even cameras. Ignorance of cultural needs are reasons that could factor much in the need to interpret behaviour of the individual resulting from, e.g. autistic individuals' particular needs which cause them stress. The stress then results in challenging behaviour. Social anxiety is a trait evidenced as challenging behaviour for people who suffer specific conditions, e.g. autism. Being put in a situation, e.g. of doing an interview or speaking in public causes them difficulties. Lack of control over decisions, as people with challenging behaviour may not be consulted or involved in making decisions due to constraints of comprehension or other strains. Being victims of bullying causes challenging behaviour as the victims tend to want to avoid any encounter with the perpetrators: for instance those who have been victims of Islamophobia or racism may avoid areas where there are less likely to be others who share their background.

- Psychological causes of challenging behaviour come from the individual's brain functions and can be any of the following, or a combination: barriers to communication, i.e. not being able to learn, commonly referred as learning disability, mental illness, or sensory impairment. Inability to process information; where the individual is unable to learn or understand, resulting into frustration, stress, and leading to behaviour that challenges. Disorientation which may be resulting from dementia and memory loss leading to failed communication and consequently behaviour that challenges. The individual suffering with behaviour that challenges could also be susceptible to depression which then causes withdrawal symptoms. As part of the example of psychological causes is "personality disorder" where the individual does not even understand the likely result of their actions. There is also the element of being "psychotic" which sets off aggressive and unprovoked outbursts, which become behaviour that challenges.

- Transitional causes of behaviour that challenges are an example too: drawing example from personal experience as a migrant British, I found the whole thing very daunting, frightening, and taxing. I felt I had lost all my friends and relatives, I had lost personal effects, and to move from one country to another. Observers seeing me traumatised may have noticed behaviour that challenged. For children, changing a school, e.g. from nursery to primary or from primary to secondary, distresses individuals. What would help is to prepare the individual, e.g. by setting up visits to the intended environment and getting to meet some of the staff and others.

- House moving is referred to as one of the most distressing happenings in life. However, preparation and understanding may help individuals who are likely to exhibit challenging behaviour. Changes in family such as a bereavement or divorce may also cause behaviour that challenges. The individual needs to transit from what they were used to in order to accept the new. Changes for individuals who are autistic is a cause for distress and I draw from my own child who is in this condition; the smell of food or the change of clothes' colour, the loss of friends or people she is used to due to school transition causes challenging behaviour unless she is sat down and prepared for a period. There is a dislike of suddenness.

- Learned behaviour that challenges is possible resulting from the company of those around an individual. Human beings begin to accept that when they do A then B may follow. Actions provoking reactions; if one is hit, they respond by either hitting back or running away: learning from others is a major factor especially with children. Tantrums are usually started by a sibling and the others copy it. A child seeking attention, by shouting; then, other children also begin to learn that when that child shouted they got what they wanted, so the others learn it; although it may not be the appropriate thing to do, it could develop into a habit if not understood and contained appropriately. Learning the consequences of behaviour is very important for children, young people, and adults so that bad behaviour is not rewarded, hence governments put up correctional institutions and the law deals with lawlessness at the extreme end of behaviour. However with children a treat should be a reward for good behaviour. When challenging behaviour is shown, a child should be calmed down and spoken to calmly to ensure they do not learn behaviour that challenges.

CHAPTER 3

The challenge posed by the impact of challenging behaviour

AN EXPLANATION OF THE IMPACT AND EFFECTS OF CHALLENGING BEHAVIOUR ON THE CLIENT WHO COULD BE A CHILD OR AN ADULT INDIVIDUAL:

The following is an explanation of impact and effects of behaviour that challenges on individuals:

It is additional to understanding and negative attitudes: there are mainly four main aspects in which behaviours that challenge impact on the individual:

(a) Social: Society has an impact on us. Socially an individual can become popular, labelled, or stigmatised. This makes a base to grow behaviour that challenges. A person affected can then begin to unfriend formerly good relations, break family ties, walk away from society or groups that were once good friends.

(b) Emotionally: Emotions result from how we feel. My child who has a diagnosis of autism and learning disability has awareness that she has this condition and that she sometimes has the ability to do certain things well and others poorly. She is aware that she has no power or control to circumnavigate the situation; what she has done positively is to devise or learn survival skills. It is common for individuals to be embarrassed, hence refuse to socialise or isolate themselves due to feeling shame or feel intimidated by those who are more able. In other cases individuals have behaviour that challenges without knowing it. There are cases of the individual not having the ability to interpret or comprehend social cues. The effects of behaviour that challenges make individuals require support to be understood and cope with situations. Guilt is common; people who fail to understand social cues may feel guilty complexes leading to behaviour that challenges with emotional impact. Observation of the individual and understanding why is critical for carers so that emotions are not misplaced, misinterpreted, in order to reassure the individual.

(c) Physical: Well-being is the key for the carer to ensure that an individual who has particular physical injuries is mentally well. When behaviour that challenges begins to be displayed in psychological format there are evidences to look out for such as an individual self-harming by:
- Burning or subjecting themselves to fire injury
- Bruising, e.g. individuals head-banging on walls
- Bites, self-biting, even as simple as lip biting or nail biting
- Cuts; where for instance wrists have been slashed as a result of self-hate
- Head injuries that are self-inflicted
- Scratches, where there is no itching but simply to self-injure as a result of self-hate

Those are effects of the impact of the behaviour that challenges, when appropriately observed and understood in context.

(d) Psychological: The explanation of impact and effects of behaviour that challenges in the individual is also seen as psychological in three ways:

1. Avoidance: wherein the individual avoids what may be necessary or even good, e.g. medication.

2. Reward; wherein the individual repeatedly seeks pleasure in the enjoyment of what they got after a behaviour or act.

3. Response or reaction; wherein the individual gets pleasure when responded to for their actions, e.g. a baby cries and gets milk.

The above are the effects of the impact of behaviour that challenges. Therefore, individuals' conduct or behaviour are different and also have different impacts on them and society, therefore, as a carer or care worker I or you must be aware that as I or you deal with any behaviour that challenges, there is no reduction in the quality of life of the individual I or you care for. For example do all it takes, e.g. the child that has a behaviour to refuse food needs supplements to ensure that they do not deteriorate in weight and growth.

That is how any carer can and you should explain the impact of behaviour that challenges on an individual and the carer.

CHAPTER 4

The challenge of understanding how to support positive behaviour

HOW TO IDENTIFY WHEN AN INDIVIDUAL'S BEHAVIOUR MAY ESCALATE

Explaining how to recognise changes in individuals that may indicate an episode of challenging behaviour:

How to recognise changes in a child or an individual that may indicate an episode of challenging behaviour requires you, the care worker, to have knowledge: knowledge is power. In order to be in control of any given situation demands knowledge. A good knowledge of background information of the "individual/sufferer" of challenging behaviour is the key to recognising changes in a child or an individual that may indicate an episode of challenging behaviour. This is an explanation of how to recognise changes in individuals that may indicate an episode of behaviour that challenges: any recognition comes about through knowledge or information: the care worker must be informed and thereby knowledgeable.

This book teaches you as care workers to be able to recognise changes in an individual's behaviour which may give an indication of the occurrence of behaviour that challenges. The indication can be defined as indicators or triggers. How a care worker may recognise these indicators requires action that methodically and accurately understands the individual who is likely to have behaviour that challenges. As carer I would read on any notes or particular file of the individual in order to know; there would be a carer plan on that file which should give indication of the indicators/triggers that cause them to behave challengingly. As care worker I would have to find out about the individual, by visiting them; visit and interact with their close relations such as family or any friends: it would be important to get a briefing or make references with others such as social workers or doctors, generally other professionals working with the individual, so that the "how" question is addressed to enable recognition of changes in an individual that would indicate likely episodes of behaviour that challenges and how to deal with it. Through this, three good things would become available to the care worker:

1. This would facilitate required information to know how to recognise changes in the individual that may indicate behaviour that challenges. E.g. in my childcare facility we have a policy for the allocated staff that would be "key worker" for a pre-school child to make a home visit prior to the start date for the child, but following admission to the facility. This way the worker gets to know the child, the parents, and the environment the child resides in. If necessary, a couple of visits to interact with the child in the presence of parents. This helps prevent anxiety for the child, but also reassures the parents when the child eventually comes into the childcare facility. Therefore, a good knowledge of background information of the "individual/sufferer" of challenging behaviour is the key to recognising changes in a child or an individual that may indicate an episode of behaviour that challenges.

2. How to deal with the individual or respond positively to support or help the individual: e.g. there have been instances of children with low sugar needs requiring the administration of

insulin at the childcare facility I am involved with: the staff are able to respond to these needs by having had prior contact and information through familiarisation visits to the homes and consultation with the nurses that care for any individual child in this category. A good knowledge of background information of the "individual/sufferer" of challenging behaviour is the key to recognising changes in a child or an individual that may indicate an episode of behaviour that challenges.

3. How the carer or care worker would ensure self-safety, the safety of others, and the safety of the individual. When the carer is equipped with a good knowledge of background information of the "individual/sufferer" of challenging behaviour they then have the "how-to" key to recognising changes in a child or an individual that may indicate an episode of behaviour that challenges, if for instance the worker needs to use protective gloves for likely fluid expel or there is a need to call in a co-worker to assist with restraint.

Therefore, we conclude that a good knowledge of background information of the "individual/sufferer" of challenging behaviour is the "how" or key to recognising changes in a child or an individual that may indicate an episode of behaviour that challenges.

This chapter gives a carer an excellent scope to understand, having reflected upon own practice. We are certainly right to say that one would find out about the child or individual and identify a wide range of people who one might speak to in order to do this. A friend whose own practice as a social worker supporting young people with autism often contacts or makes referrals for advocacy support for the person she is supporting. Often young people with learning disabilities and autism lack the mental capacity to make informed decisions about things like their care and support. By including an advocate you get an independent view of what the person's wishes and feelings would be.

CHAPTER 5

Understanding how to support positive behaviour

THE CHALLENGE OF THE IMPORTANCE OF IDENTIFYING PATTERNS OF BEHAVIOUR AND TRIGGERS TO CHALLENGING BEHAVIOUR:

Here we make reference to at least two types of behaviour:

It is important to identify the patterns of behaviour and triggers to behaviour that challenges. In this answer I refer to some types of behaviour:

Identifying patterns of behaviour that challenges:

This is when the carer recognises changes or actions in an individual. The changes recognised would be indicative of likely episodes of challenging behaviour.

Triggers to behaviour that challenges:

The triggers that the carer should recognise are the ways or pointers of behaviour; that the individual cared for is about to become, e.g. aggressive, have a fit, etc.

1). TRIGGERS:

They are the cause. They cause other things to occur. The trigger "thirst" causes the desire for drink. The way to recognise changes that an individual is leading towards episodes of challenging behaviour is to ensure that carers and others concerned with the welfare of the individual are aware of these pointers or triggers that cause or exacerbate behaviour that challenges. It is important to safeguard against triggers; for instance in this case we can take an example of how honey attracts bees, yet the bees produce the honey, so when honey is taken and left in any open place, somehow bees come hunting or towards that honey: it is, therefore, important to discern if consistency is rife when challenging behaviour takes place in an individual or is it dependent on time factors, conditions, or mood. As everyone is different so factors of triggers for each individual are different. It is therefore relevant that each individual is known and that whatever their trigger for behaviour that challenges is, is recognised and known. When the carer knows the likely trigger for the sufferer, then appropriate responses can be made. It is just like if someone has whooping cough, that cough triggers vomiting and the carer would do well to provide an inhaler for breathing ease and a basin to catch the likely sick.

Triggers are similar to irritation: I suffer from hay fever and whilst I find the colours of flowers pleasant to see, the pollen makes me itch and suffer uncontrollable sneezing unless I take the precaution of taking medication antihistamines. The carer therefore is duty-bound to ensure background knowledge of individuals in order to know what triggers challenging behaviour.

There are numerous behavioural challenge triggers, among them environmental and circumstantial triggers:

- Environmental triggers: These include things like lighting, noise, darkness, heat, cold, crowds, or congestion.

- Circumstantial triggers: These are more to do with feelings of the individual such as thirst, tiredness, hunger, or toileting. Circumstances will also include unwanted focus of individuals or unwanted attention. They include withdrawal of things from the individual, e.g. if the individual smokes the stoppage or withdrawal of the cigarettes can trigger behaviour that challenges. It is also common if food that is disliked is given to the individual with challenging behaviour that the behaviour is aggravated.

Social triggers; in society, e.g. in a school community, teasing or being bullied can trigger behaviour that challenges, and oftentimes children will pick on someone who looks different. Some instances occur when the individual with challenging behaviour is put in an awkward position of speaking or talking to someone who they do not wish to interact with or talk to.

- Health triggers can occur and cause challenging behaviour due to such examples as being made to do things that are seemingly of no value but ritual. Mental health problems can be a trigger to behaviour that challenges, then medication side effects and being in pain, suffering debilitation, or feeling oppressed.

It is, therefore, important to identify the patterns of behaviour and triggers to behaviour that challenges.

2. TECHNIQUES OF AVOIDANCE:

It is important to identify the patterns of behaviour and triggers to behaviour that challenges as this enables the carer to take appropriate action: one such action is techniques of avoidance. Without knowing the patient's history or background to what triggers their challenging behaviour the carer would not be able to employ "avoidance techniques". Equipped with the care plan, the carer can use five of the known avoidance techniques in order to control triggers or render them ineffective:

a). Communication: This can be used in various ways to control triggers; the manner or method of communicating with the individual can be changed or altered: where frustration or anxiety is identified when communication is made, changes can be made. For instance, people who are bilingual may be more comfortable speaking in another language. This is critical information to be on the care plan. Family and friends or social workers can help in ensuring that a particular manner of communication is listed. In my childcare setting we receive children who require Makaton and sign language because they are non-verbal, but we also have children from bilingual communities or those new to Britain and we have to devise the various communication methods including volunteer language teachers to support the individual. Therefore, it is important to identify the patterns of behaviour and triggers to behaviour that challenges.

b). Praise for good: In my nursery setting, praising children and staff is critical to achieving desired outcomes. Therefore, to control triggers of challenging behaviour for an individual it is important the carer uses the avoidance of such behaviour by throwing in the "praise" where good actions are evidenced. Praise can take the shape of words or reward. Therefore, it is important to identify the patterns of behaviour and triggers to behaviour that challenges.

c). Altering the environment: It is important to know the background of the individual and some instances call for environmental changes to control behaviour that challenges. If a baby cannot sleep, maybe the room is too cold or too hot. But also things like confinement can cause individuals to feel claustrophobic and a simple controlled or supervised walk can help with avoidance of triggers of behaviour that challenges. Therefore, it is important to identify the patterns of behaviour and triggers to behaviour that challenges.

d). Techniques of distraction: These can vary but are important to use once the carers identify the patterns of behaviour and triggers to behaviour that challenges in an individual. It can be a promise that can be kept; in my nursery we can promise that "…we will go home at the close of school if we all behave well." If it is pizza day for lunch there is no harm in saying that "If we all listen carefully, we will have our pizza at lunch time." The distraction has to be good to do the trick of persuading the individual not to be triggered into challenging behaviour. The distraction is always an alternative or preference. It is important to identify the patterns of behaviour and triggers to behaviour that challenges.

e). Induction or preparation: The technique of avoiding triggers of behaviour that challenges can be helped by avoiding sudden changes. Therefore the carers must know that it is important to identify the patterns of behaviour and triggers to behaviour that challenges in order to employ avoidance by induction or preparation of the individual to changes. When young children are due to move into a new school, it helps if they are taken to that school to meet the would-be new teacher and to see what rooms they will be in. This technique helps the individual not to focus on triggers of fear of the unknown.

3). TYPES OF TRIGGERS THAT MAY CAUSE AN INDIVIDUAL TO HAVE CHALLENGING BEHAVIOUR:

For the carer to determine what type of behaviour is being triggered, the importance of identifying the patterns of behaviour and triggers to behaviour that challenges becomes critical for the appropriate response.

a). New behaviour that is identifiable: I start with this point as it can happen to any one individual and can occur at any time. It could be a new carer walking into the room if transition was not done, or a piece of cloth that is undesired, etc. The "something else or unknown" not on the file or the care plan of an individual may trigger challenging behaviour. It may be something that is concealed or hidden. The carer has a duty to be able to identify what is the cause of behaviour. However, new triggers are a type of trigger. It is important to identify the patterns of behaviour and triggers to behaviour that challenges.

b). Seeking attention: Seeking attention can be an identifiable habit: individuals could exhibit challenging behaviour in order to draw attention to themselves or to an issue or situation around themselves. Boredom plays significantly in situations where individuals show challenging behaviour. Usually engagement and distractions can help in alleviating the problem; but then again it is attention the individual wanted. However always carers must investigate if the trigger was attention seeking or something else, never drawing conclusions prior to investigation. It is important, therefore, to identify the patterns of behaviour and triggers to behaviour that challenges.

c). Ritualistic: Ritualistic behaviour happens for various reasons: when individuals with challenging behaviour get anxiety or may become bored, and in many cases lack stimuli, they then get triggered into the ritual; such as crying for no reason, rocking from side to side, screaming, or pulling at their hair or clothing, etc. In some cases if the individual has sensory problems they may also exhibit some of those traits. My child with autism and sensory issues normally spins around with hands stretched; one time in an airport she hit a lady passing close to her with no intention, but because she was spinning as she was finding the travelling and rodomontade of airport routines boring. Thus, it is important to identify the patterns of behaviour and triggers to behaviour that challenges.

d). Learned triggers: Lessons are learned by individuals with challenging behaviour, as they adopt issues and associate those issues with the habit. Music can be a sign for dancing, but certain types of music could signal going to sleep. Reward for good behaviour is often used by carers in situations where challenging behaviour is being dealt with. Therefore, it is important to identify the patterns of behaviour and triggers to behaviour that challenges.

e). Avoidance behaviour is identifiable. Since carers know the individual, they will know from the care plan that the individual does not like going to the doctor; the individual may have learned that to go to the doctor may earn them an injection or other unpleasant treatment for their condition. Therefore when such times occur, there may be resistance as an expression of avoidance. Avoidant behaviour can include things like running away. Children with autism and hearing issues or sensory issues run away on hearing certain noises, e.g. fire engine or ambulance and police sirens. They are trying to avoid the situation. So it is important to identify the patterns of behaviour and triggers to behaviour that challenges.

f). Routine behaviour can be identified: It is important for the carer to identify the patterns of behaviour and triggers to behaviour that challenges. Routine is the manner of things done and that frequently happen at the specific instance. Behaviour that challenges is consistent and specific. My child with autism always tells me she does not like change. She resists new things or places, she wants what she knows and what she is used to, yet she has a mind and ability to recognise that she does not like change and can say so. For the carer it is therefore very important to identify the patterns of behaviour and triggers to behaviour that challenges.

4). OBSERVATIONS DONE OBJECTIVELY:

In order for carers to identify the patterns of behaviour and triggers to behaviour that challenges, they must carry out objective observations of individuals who have challenging behaviour and ensure objective development of coping strategies: the care worker can then equip oneself with avoidant or survival strategies. The care plan and updates made on it are notes resulting from objective observations. The carer does not need to calculate why behaviour is challenging, but the duty is to record the reality of the apparent. Not making assumptions but recording what reality is and happening. This course helps the carer to ensure that no stereotypes or labels are made of the individual with behaviour that challenges. There are six strategies of identifying patterns of behaviour to arrive at an objective observation:

i). The behaviours that are seen or observed

ii). The people/others present

iii). What happened where intervention was impossible?

iv). The things that occur prior to the trigger of challenging behaviour

v). Is there a record of similar occurrences/incidents?

vi). Where did the incident occur?

The carer would do well to record any of the above observations in an objective manner for instance if the child or individual gets agitated every time there is a visitor unknown to the child or individual, etc.

Therefore, objective observations of individuals and the development of coping strategies are important to identify the patterns of behaviour and triggers to behaviour that challenges.

5). UNKNOWN TRIGGERS:

Life is a mystery. It is impossible to know everything. This is why it is important for carers to identify the patterns of behaviour and triggers to behaviour that challenges. However, when new triggers are causing challenging behaviour, those new triggers may not be known and not on the file or care plan of an individual. Therefore observations must be objective, but in instances where objective observations do not identify the trigger, then extra measures such as consulting other professionals, family members, and others who have a link with the individual may be invaluable sources of identifying that trigger. Further observations must continue in the effort to establish the trigger. Strategic observation plans must be implemented and maybe over a period the trigger may be identified. Therefore, even in cases of unknown triggers it is important to identify the patterns of behaviour which ultimately help in identifying triggers to behaviour that challenges.

6). RECORDING BEHAVIOURAL PATTERNS:

It is important to record the patterns of behaviour: thereby, capturing events and issues that identify the patterns of behaviour and triggers to challenging behaviour. It is important to follow a way that is recognisable by carers in recording so that information can be shared where appropriate and in order to improve the quality of the individual. The records are a point of reference at all times. This book teaches us to use the following structure:

i) The method of video recording: what I have found best to use is video recording in care if this does not infringe the rights of the individual:

- Advantages of video recording include that it records if specific issues or behaviour happen in a particular place or instance. Advantageous is also the fact that verbal and non-verbal behaviour get recorded and can be observed at review. Advantage is there so interactions or communications made with others or with the carer are easy to define. Video recording therefore helps in enhancing the fact that it is important to identify the patterns of behaviour and triggers to behaviour that challenges.

- There are disadvantages though in using video recording: these include the unpredictability of circumstances; behaviour can change when an obvious method of recording is being used. There is also a disadvantage if lighting or noise suddenly interferes with the capturing of incidents. Most disadvantageous, video recording requires equipment and an operator even if these were phones, cameras, or CCTV. However we have learnt that it is important to record any identified patterns of behaviour and triggers to behaviour that challenges.

ii) Written method:

Use written notes. These can be in handwriting or typed format.

- Advantages:

The advantages of written notes include being convenient and that they can be done very fast, can be referred to quickly, can be done discreetly, and can be done without using special equipment.

- Disadvantages:

There are disadvantages of written notes, for instance if the writing was not immediate, some issues or events may be left out due to forgetting or memory lapse. Also some things could be missed out when writing. Notes can also be difficult to include or make detailed observations in.

However, the method of taking notes helps us record and reference for it is important to identify the patterns of behaviour and triggers to behaviour that challenges.

iii) Audio recorded method:

- The advantages here are that: through the audio recording, the carer can capture the verbal interactions with the individual.

Advantages also include the fact that usually nothing is missed, when and how it was said and by who. There is advantage for the carer as carers can then listen for specific tones and words as they were used. Such audio recordings can be done secretly.

- The disadvantages of audio recording of events include that: their effectiveness is impaired if the surrounding had other noises or interference. Audio can also miss out the events or issues that were non-verbal, for instance facial expressions or gestures. Audio recording can be disadvantageous as the carer would need equipment and equipment may sometimes require more than one individual caring or tending to the individual with challenging behaviour whilst another operated the equipment.

THE PROFESSIONAL TECHNIQUES OR WAYS OF RECORDING OR CAPTURING BEHAVIOUR:

The importance of identifying the patterns of behaviour and triggers to behaviour that **challenges is supported by ways of capturing behaviour that is observed. This course helps to articulate the techniques of understanding of capturing specific behaviour:**

i). Anecdotal ways; which are planned in advance or sudden with spontaneity can be of immense benefit especially with new unexpected behaviour exhibits. It is a narrative or storytelling method as the story happens. The story is done simultaneously as the observation: you see it and say/tell it as it is.

ii). Timing specific events technique: Observations that are timed for specified times or sessions of care can help in the quality of life of the individual if; new or specific identified triggers: the advantage is being able to put a time and place to the event, and incidents. I have encouraged the use of CCTV in childcare settings as then parents would be able to see on review how any anecdotal incidents may have been observed or taken place.

iii). Event technique: This is about the observation that is linked to particular events or incidents: my child that has sensory issues with autism always will want to run to her bedroom if any cooking is being done. For some reason the event of cooking smells is undesirable, yet if cooking finishes and food is served she will turn up to eat and enjoy it. We have learnt that the steaming and smoking of food is an undesirable for her. Therefore observation based on event or activity can help in defining the patterns of reaction or behaviour.

iv). Targeted individual: The issue of transition preparation always helps familiarise individuals with what's next, what to expect. But individuals can encounter strangers and in cases of individuals with behaviour that challenges, there are some cases where an individual is aggressive for meeting or encountering certain people. It is as if the individual's trigger is provoked by the presence of the other person. The technique of recording an observation that is targeted with an individual helps to identify the trigger for it is important to identify the patterns of behaviour and triggers to behaviour that challenges.

A description of why it is important to support children or individuals to recognise their limitations and take avoidance actions:

In the care service it is important to identify when an individual's behaviour may escalate: to identify such, it is critical that care workers know how to support their clients to be able to recognise their limitations and build in care services avoidance measures or action:

The limitations and what they are:
Limitations are evidenced when one cannot cope beyond a certain capacity: maximum capacity or potential is the end of the line, and when an individual cannot cope anymore and there is more that can be done or achieved, then a limit has been reached. Individuals with behaviour that challenges sometimes get to the limit when the environment becomes unbearable and they cannot cope anymore. Usually there are warning signs that a limit has been reached and the individual's behaviour may escalate.

There are warning signs to show that a limitation has been reached:
Noticeable changes or warning signs, commonly identified as triggers, begin to show, this being a clear indication the individual has reached a limit and their behaviour is going to change negatively. The change could be detrimental if action is not taken. Carers are equipped to take avoidant action, e.g. a distraction or an anti-stress measure. It is important to identify the patterns of behaviour and triggers to behaviour that challenges. Warning signs could either be very obvious or even subtle; also verbal or non-verbal expressions can be detected in observation of an individual. Therefore, in care it is important to identify when an individual's behaviour may escalate: to identify such, it is critical that care workers know how to support their clients to be able to recognise their limitations and build in care services avoidance measures or action:

Identifying Warning Signs:
The care worker has to be on guard, be alert, because in care it is important to identify when an individual's behaviour may escalate: when the behaviour escalates and the warning signs are not taken into account, or action is delayed, the individual may escalate into:

- Self-harm or harming others
- Damaging property or equipment
- Smashing and throwing things
- Physical and verbal assaults of others

To identify such warning signs, it is critical that care workers know how to support their clients to be able to recognise their limitations and build in care services avoidance measures or action. The early warning signs which show that an individual is taking a turn for the worst may range from any of the following:

- Becoming restless and panic

- Becoming argumentative

- Rapid breathing

- Flaring nostrils

- Threatening behaviour

- Shuddering or shaking

- Repetitive movement

- Reddening in the face

- Sweating

- Verbal abuse and swearing

- Clenching of fists and flexing of muscle

- Sudden outbursts including swearing

- Anger and aggression

These behavioural warnings indicate that behaviour is about to escalate; so in care it is important to identify when an individual's behaviour may escalate: to identify such warning signs it is critical that care workers know how to support their clients to be able to recognise their limitations and build in care services avoidance measures or action. The action may be to draw or develop a behaviour support plan to support behaviour that challenges, or implement such a plan if one is already in existence.

Developing behavioural support plans for challenging behaviour:

Using of a documented behaviour support plan to support behaviour that challenges is a very important tool because in care it is important to identify when an individual's behaviour may escalate: to identify such, it is critical that care workers know how to support their clients to be able to recognise their limitations and build in care services avoidance measures or action. A behaviour support plan is put in place where appropriately an individual receives care, particularly for individuals with challenging behaviour as a trait. This document may be or can be part of the care plan. Such a document enables carers to reference what can be done for the client at a particular time and when certain behaviour warning signs are shown. In all situations the behaviour support plan must contain the following information:

- Name and age of the individual

- Any conditions that need tending to by the carer

- Medicines and their side effects as appropriate

- Methods of medicine administration as preferred by the client

- What triggers challenging behaviour; the warning signs

- How the individual manages their own behaviour; calming applications

- How the individual can be calmed

- Emergency contacts when incidents occur, e.g. relatives, friends, professionals

Therefore, in the care industry it is important to identify when an individual's behaviour may escalate: to identify such, it is critical that care workers know how to support their clients to be able to recognise their limitations and build in care services avoidance measures or action using what information has been placed on a "behavioural support plan".

Application of diversion techniques in supporting behaviour that challenges:

To divert the client from behaviour that is detrimental we bear in mind that in the care industry it is important to identify when an individual's behaviour may escalate: to identify such, it is critical that care workers know how to support their clients to be able to recognise their limitations and build in care services avoidance measures or action. The carer has a duty to apply measures that ensure that the quality of life of the individual is not reduced but improved. The carer must consult with the support plan to be guided as to what to do when behaviour is likely to escalate: one technique that is proven in behavioural management is the "use of diversion to support behaviour that challenges". The diversions are many and varied. Among them are:

- Reminding the client of appropriate behaviour

- Using some relaxation technique that worked previously

- Introduction of some form of physical activity which the client may have a preference for; children in a nursery may be helped into a song for instance

- Helping talk to the individual about something away or else from the focus which seems to trigger or escalate behaviour

- Going out for walks or for a run or another exercise

- Helping remove the individual from the situation

- Devising, introduction of, or offers of alternative activities

The application of diversionary techniques in supporting behaviour that challenges in caring for individuals is important to identify when an individual's behaviour may escalate: to identify such, it is critical that care workers know how to support their clients to be able to recognise their limitations and build in care services diversionary and avoidance measures or action.

CHAPTER 6

The challenge posed by strategies to support positive behaviour

The description of strategies that could be used to support positive behaviour

In order to describe strategies that could be applied to supporting positive behaviour we must understand that it is important to identify when an individual's behaviour may escalate: to identify such strategies as will support positive behaviour, it is critical that care workers know how to support their clients to be able to recognise their limitations and build in care services avoidance measures or action that would then lead to positive behaviour: the positive outcome. In the first instance it is important to understand what positive behaviour is and then enumerate the strategies that can be used to ensure positive behaviour:

Positive behaviour can be defined to include cooperating with the carer or others, sharing, e.g. information about self, communicating effectively, making sense, building positive relationships, helping as appropriate, forgiving, upholding, or having good manners and being apologetic when in the wrong. Where there is a need to use strategies that could be applied to support positive behaviour:

<u>**The strategies include:**</u>

1. The carer being consistent in approaching the behaviour that challenges: This means doing the right thing at all times in spite of the pressures around. The individual being cared for needs to get the same message. In my childcare setting I ensure that parents are informed, updated on what is being communicated to children, so that parents can also communicate the same. Clients can become confused if consistency is not applied in communication. That can intensify challenging behaviour instead of helping support the individual.

2. The carers must praise and reward positive behaviour. Complimenting individuals is appreciated and usually builds confidence. The client in the situations of challenging behaviour usually sees compliments as reward for good behaviour. In childcare we use a sticker or the star of the day system to enable children to realise that goodness is praised and rewarded. They all try hard each day to be that star of the day, hence promoting positive behaviour strategically.

3. The carer must use "role modelling of positive behaviour". Due to the nature of the carer and client relationship, clients may copy carer mannerisms. Saying thank you may be copied from teachers by learners, and children who are thanked for the good things they do learn to say thank you. The strategy to be a role model in the case of an individual with behaviour that challenges may enable that individual to say thank you as appropriate, thereby promoting positive behaviour.

4. Carers must never punish challenging behaviour: There are always improved changes in early years education. Some time back a child who stepped out of the norm would be excluded to a "naughty step/corner". Now we have improved that to "a time-out", this being that maybe the behaviour was due to the individual needing time-out, away a little bit from the main group. The idea is to show all that it is not punishing, but stepping away to adjust and re-join. This method works better than punishing. It is important that the individual understands why and how the measure or strategy is applied to them. Punishing is never understood by people with behaviour that challenges.

5. Carers must enable the individual to communicate in a way they prefer: In advancing this strategy in my childcare setting we strive to communicate with parents from various backgrounds, some of whom do not speak much English, so we have a diverse staff and pool of volunteers that speak multiple languages to enable us to demonstrate to the parents that we appreciate who they are; we speak their languages. There are non-verbal children in our special inclusion provision where Makaton and pictorial communication are used to advance this strategy.

6. Carers must have that patient/client and compassionate attitude: This strategy helps the client not to increase in agitation; when they pick up positive vibes from their carer, they have more confidence in them. When the carer is communicating well, the client feels the compassion and care from the carer. The client then will open up and freely discuss their problems.

These strategies could be applied to clients to support their positive behaviour; therefore we must understand that it is important to identify when an individual's behaviour may escalate.

Again the above description is a really good statement and it is that we have provided examples of strategies to use as an alternative from punishing the child or an individual for challenging behaviour. In childcare, using the naughty step was made widely understood through the TV show *Supernanny*. The following web link talks about strategies for younger children such as naughty step, time-out, and using rewards. Anyone in childcare work might find it interesting.

https://www.supernanny.co.uk/Advice/-/Parenting-Skills/-/Discipline-and-Reward/The-Naughty-Step-~-what-is-it-and-how-does-it-work.aspx

Describing the advantages of proactive strategies in supporting positive behaviour

1) **PROACTIVE STRATEGIES:**

There are advantages in employing proactive strategies in supporting positive behaviour. Carers should know that what has already been prepared as a strategy is what is meant by proactive strategy. These ready-made strategies could be applied to supporting positive behaviour and we must understand that it is important to identify when an individual's behaviour may escalate in order to draw on proactive strategies to calm down the individual. Carers can draw on such proactive strategies as listed here:

Carers can ensure "environmental changes": space or location, routines, or stimulants such as objects in the care environment.

Carers can "establish boundaries and set rules": whereby the client/individuals know and are aware of how far they can go, e.g. walking around the care area. E.g. children know that they are not allowed to bring sweets to school. Children know they cannot go home until home-time and the bell has rung. Individuals, once aware of the limits, act accordingly or make amendments.

Carers can provide "skills development": Carers can help individuals to acquire new skills and this helps in the reduction of showing challenging behaviours. The skill will vary according to ability. Playing a musical instrument, learning to read, or even just playing games with others using an iPad can all contribute to increased quality of life when learned as a skill by individuals that have challenging behaviour.

Provision of a quiet and safe environment: Such space is a proactive aim of childcare settings and is part of their remit. When carers are using the provision as a quiet and safe environment it helps the calming of individuals from escalating challenging behaviour. Therefore in planning housing or accommodation for the individual in need, this strategy is very much at work.

Carers should know how to observe an individual to identify triggers: To reduce the likelihood of behaviour that challenges taking place, care workers must have the knowledge of how to observe and what to look for, when and how to act in order to ascertain the triggers that are likely to be taking place and may result into an escalation for an individual.

Carers must provide focussed support: The person-centred support should be put alongside the provision of the care plan. Within the actual delivery the carer then ensures knowledge and information taken from the plan to ensure:

- Individual calming techniques

- Communication passports

- Personal/individual obstruction and calming techniques

Focussed support is brought about by the initial plan when the client is taken on, through information provided and spelling out who the individual is. Such information will be enriched by family members and/or professionals who know the likes, or who are aware of medication that the individual needs, etc.

Carers must uphold and be aware of policies and procedures: The carer that is well trained knows what procedures are followed, step by step, to ensure the outcome of positive behaviour from an individual. All workers for an individual must be acquainted with procedure look up or make references when a situation arises and triggers are seemingly evident, ensuring that the care plan is brought into play, identifying the triggers and taking avoidant action, step by step, ensuring the reduction of challenging behaviour triggers.

Carers must take account of environmental changes: Individuals with challenging behaviour could easily be affected by changes in environment. If for instance the routine the individual is used to suddenly changes, this could trigger challenging behaviour or its escalation. Individuals used to having a cup of tea first thing in the morning can have the whole day upset if they missed that occasion. To promote positive behaviour such routines must be maintained.

There are advantages in employing proactive strategies in supporting positive behaviour. Carers should know that what has already been prepared as a strategy is what is meant by proactive strategy.

2) CARERS SHOULD KNOW THAT PROACTIVE STRATEGIES IMPACT ON AN INDIVIDUAL:

In care, positive outcomes are essential for the individual. Carers must know that proactive strategies can produce those positive outcomes and reduce the likelihood of escalation in challenging behaviour. Carers should know that what has already been prepared as a strategy is what is meant by proactive strategy. When carers consistently use proactive strategies the care becomes consistent and this is achieved through the following eight proactive strategies:

i. Positive social interactions increase: The company of an individual who has now shown positive behaviour normally will be friendly and others will want to be in their company. On the contrary, when challenging behaviour is evident many people do not wish to be in the company of the individual showing it. When the individual is aggressive others are scared or put off from interacting.

When individuals have no positive social interaction they are either scary or frightened. Therefore, carers should know that what has already been prepared as a strategy is what is meant by proactive strategy.

ii. Increasing in confidence and self-esteem: When positive behaviour is prompted, it is through the carers knowing that what has already been prepared as a strategy is what is meant by proactive strategy: the carer prompts the individual to increase in confidence and esteem by complimenting, reassuring them to interact. Environment and routine can be brought into the equation by for instance inviting other people to visit the individual in the comfort of their home or at meal times and eat together.

Therefore, carers should know that what has already been prepared as a strategy is what is meant by proactive strategy and this helps in management of triggers and prevention of onset of challenging behaviour.

iii. Family and friends' satisfaction is increased: The goodness and overall improvement in health is a positive impact and helps the individual to respond positively to relations such as friends and family, even to the professionals themselves. Once the client is behaviourally calm and settled the positive effects are felt all round. Relatives are no longer worried or tense, the individual interacts more, and there is an air of overall increase in satisfaction for family and friends. This would be the result of carers implementing the knowledge that what has already been prepared as a strategy is what is meant by proactive strategy.

iv. Reduction in challenging behaviour: Proactive strategies impact tremendously in the reduction of challenging behaviour when carers know that what has already been prepared as a strategy is what is meant by proactive strategy and implement it positively. Reduction of behaviour that challenges is the aim of the carer; it is the ultimate achievement when positive behaviour occurs in an individual. The combination of all strategies in a consistent manner following policies will benefit the individual; this is when the individual's support plan will be executed.

v. Increasing collaboration with care workers: This is a clear goal and aspiration, and is achievable; when the strategies devised and developed are implemented in the care plan for an individual, care workers generate satisfaction and relief. This way engenders best practice and joint responses to behaviour that challenges: this impact or situation comes about when the combination of strategies: care workers will increase their collaboration for the individual and others in their care, building a strong team that cares and achieves goals through proactive strategies.

vi. Increased trust in others: Once self-esteem and confidence in oneself is rekindled in the individual with challenging behaviour, trust in others is restored, positive behaviour happens: this is positive impact and happens where the consistency of care has been employed by carers who collaborate and work as a team using proactive strategies. Carers too begin to trust the individual and can allow interaction with others. Carers can now predict or expect positive behaviour. The individual can also predict their own triggers and express concern to the carer. These things happen as a result of carers knowing that what has already been prepared as a strategy is what is meant by proactive strategy and this helps in management of triggers and prevention of onset of challenging behaviour. The trust secured in the individual will help in increasing collaboration with care workers and the carers will trust and expect positive behaviour from the individual.

vii. Increase in the well-being overall: To be a whole person and realise full potential or work towards it requires overall well-being. When the individual begins to trust and be trusted, when family and friends find satisfaction in being with the individual among other positive things, the individual will begin to show signs of well-being. Well-being of an individual reduces challenging behaviour. Increased well-being will come about to contribute to mental and physical wellness. Carers can help the well-being of an individual to impact positive behaviour by implementing knowledge that what has already been prepared as a strategy is what is meant by proactive strategy and this helps in management of triggers and prevention of onset of challenging behaviour.

viii. Increase in critical skills: Critical skills help individuals to discern between right and wrong. Individuals that have challenging behaviour may not be able to make discernment; they may not have the capacity to refuse or accept situations without support. The impact of proactive strategies on behaviour can help stop triggers. When triggers are arrested, the individual will not escalate. Where the escalation is managed then that individual may begin to cooperate, and make critical and objective responses to care. We teach children in nursery how to wait or take turns at play or any learning activity; through this way, carers promote positive and critical behaviour. Critical behaviour being restored or developing in an individual with behaviour that challenges is evidence that the combination of all strategies in a consistent manner following policies and implementing the care plan does benefit the individual; this is when the individual's support plan will be executed and they begin to recover towards well-being, dealing or responding to triggers: proactive strategy therefore is in place and carers are aware of it to draw on before the trigger occurs.

Again this element of the book is excellent and covers every part of the issue. Here we include a web link for a fact sheet for the use of proactive and reactive strategies to support positive behaviour. Any practitioner carer might find it useful to refer to within your practice.

http://www.challengingbehaviour.org.uk/learning-disability-files/03---Positive-Behaviour-Support-Planning-Part-3-web-2014.pdf

An explanation of the impact made through reactive strategies when supporting positive behaviour.

The reactive strategies in supporting positive behaviour can be explained in two categories, namely:

1. **Positive reactive strategies and 2. Negative reactive strategies.**

Positive reactive strategies:

The impact of reactive strategies in supporting positive behaviour is that response by carers to the individual's escalating situation. The behaviour is taking place and the carer is striving strategically to control the situation by implementing the reactive strategies. It is reactive strategies that can ensure the continued safety of the individual and those around them. We safeguard children in nursery, we ensure all precautions are taken, but then the unforeseen happens, a child falls and grazes a leg; the reactive strategy is to help the child up, examine the graze, call a colleague and ensure other children are safe, follow the injuries procedure, and the child or individual will now be anxious and distressed. In this course we learn that there are several positive reactive strategies that can be drawn from, including distraction techniques, ignoring the behaviour, use of knowledge to effectively resolve an incident of conflict, removal from the environment, supporting individuals to agree to positive resolutions when there is conflict with others, removal from an environment, ignoring the behaviour, using of distraction techniques, and using agreed physical interventions. The positive reactive strategies can only be used as a result of carers knowing that what has already been prepared as a strategy is what is meant by proactive strategy and this helps in management of triggers and prevention of onset of challenging behaviour. However, when the situation dictates, then positive reactive strategies can be the alternative to proactive strategies.

There are two categories of "reactive strategies", the positive and negative. I will explain the positive in this first instance:

(CATEGORY 1) Detail on reactive strategies:

i. Distractions: Using distraction techniques will sway the attention of the individual from focussing on the triggers causing the challenging behaviour. In ensuring that the individual is distracted, the carer manages the challenging behaviour towards more positive behaviour. Therefore reactive strategies have a great and very useful impact in supporting positive behaviour. It is important to mention that the reactive strategy is a final resort, when a carer is taken by surprise, the fall-back-on strategy is the reactive remedy. A situation arises and the carer cannot talk to the individual; a carer can show the individual a distraction, e.g. mention the individual will be taken to the cinema, if they like the cinema; the distraction works and positive behaviour happens.

ii. Ignoring the behaviour: I try this many times with my own children. When we disagree on something they have a tendency to keep talking about it, e.g. they want to buy ice cream when not appropriate, I tell them it is not appropriate, but they carry on saying how they should buy ice cream. My solution becomes to silently ignore the request and eventually they give up. This study suggests that unwanted behaviour can be extinguished by ignoring it as long as no one is being or likely to be harmed.

iii. Removal from an environment: In childcare two children sitting together can be made difficult and they can just not settle when next to each other; the solution is to separate them, partner them with others. In the care of individuals with behaviour that challenges if the individual is removed from an environment which triggers behaviour that challenges, reactively that is a good reactive strategy.

iv. Using agreed physical interventions: The safety of an individual with behaviour that challenges is critical, alongside that of others including the carers. Ensuring that the dignity of the individual is upheld, ensuring that the individual is not hurt deliberately, and in line with the support plan: there is always guidance and a procedural plan on reactive strategies of physical intervention. It is professional to ensure that strategies are in place to deal with the individual and bring them to a well-being of full potential, however, if the strategies in place have not worked or if the onset of behaviour that challenges escalated and the strategies in place are exhausted and the individual cannot be calmed down, but continues to run wild or threatens the safety of others, it is appropriate to use reactive strategies, drawing from training and learned skills, like sounding the alarm to get agreed and procedural measures to restrain the individual.

v. Care workers using knowledge effectively to resolve incidents and conflicts: The care plan usually gives the history of the individual's condition, what triggers cause them to be of challenging behaviour. Such knowledge is gathered at the start of care for the individual: this knowledge is used to either calm down the individual or bring them to the positive behaviour. Defusing any conflict or incidents of escalating challenging behaviour is possible using a reactive strategy of "using knowledge".

vi. Supporting individuals to agree to positive resolutions when there is conflict with others: Supporting individuals to do things for themselves is part of ensuring the road to recovery to full potential: individuals who can grasp messages, verbal or written, who can understand and communicate, can be supported to deal with issues and get resolutions. Therefore one of the reactive strategies to use is "supporting the individual agreeing to resolutions to situations".

(CATEGORY 2) As indicated earlier, there are two categories of "reactive strategies", the positive and negative. Having explained the positive reactions above, I will now explain the negative in this second instance:

These are the negative reactive strategies:

We should be aware and learn that at times reactive strategies may not be harnessed in a person-centred manner. In as much as the aim is to ensure the well-being of the individual. Observers of care refer to negative strategies as punitive and can include segregation and safe custody; such actions are only reactive and termed negative reactive strategies and can only be a last resort, when the individual fails to comply with support of carers to manage behaviour that challenges:

i. Medication inappropriately used: The misuse of medication by individuals with challenging behaviour can cause situations that necessitate the punitive actions as negative reaction, including admission into hospital. It is important to note that medication must always be used under professional guidance or supervision, following instructions of the prescription.

ii. Physical restraint inappropriately used: Many times, restraining individuals causes them humiliation and loss of esteem. There are several incidents in prisons and in mental health rehabilitation units where individuals have in the past been restrained and harm has come to them. However, there is particular training provision to carers who carry out such work. This work is carried out under strict guidelines and supervision. It is in such circumstances that reactive strategies may not be harnessed in a person-centred manner. The individual would be refusing support towards positive behaviour, that individual would be violent towards others, and most likely the individual would be escalating towards self-harm. Therefore the physical restraint as a reactive negative strategy is not used to harm, and not to punish or humiliate the individual, but to manage and support positive behaviour to contain behaviour that challenges.

iii. Verbally abusing and humiliating the individual: It is unacceptable and unprofessional to verbally abuse or humiliate in any way the individual suffering behaviour that challenges. This method could in reality escalate the behaviour. Knowing that the individual:

- Has no self-control

- Has no sense of understanding what is going on

- Needs help

- Needs support

Therefore, it is important that carers know what they are doing and never lose self-control, but call for help, support, and assistance from colleagues and professionals so that if used, reactive strategies may not be harnessed in a person-centred manner.

iv. Organisational cultural behaviour: Copying of behaviour is not only by individuals who suffer challenging behaviour. In organisations, certain habits or mannerisms may become traditional and may never be challenged or asked about. This can have a negative impact on organisations or cultural ways. There has been much outcry on the issue of FGM (female genital mutilation), a tradition that had gone unchallenged in some cultures for generations, and some in those communities had assumed that that is how things were meant to be. Therefore, reactive strategies may not be harnessed in a person-centred manner to support behaviour and must never be used as a way of tradition or organisational behaviour, but only in a professional way.

Reactive strategies make an impact:

When using positive reactive strategies, the role of the carer is to bring about safety from either self-harm or harm to others by the individual. The carer uses the strategies to ensure control in a situation of behaviour that challenges. Positive reactive strategies make an impact to enable carers to support the individual towards positive behaviour. When appropriately applied the individual may stabilise positively. Impact made by reactive strategies goes beyond the carer and individual and may also impact on friends and families and the society. For instance positive reactive strategies used on an individual could result in harm and this is undesirable. The negative reactive strategies, if applied and they result in harm, make society question the procedures, and confidence in care is on trial. Therefore, the impact of reactive strategies in supporting positive behaviour is that response by carers to the individual's escalating situation is managed. The behaviour is taking place and the carer is striving strategically to control the situation by implementing the reactive strategies.

There is good reference to both positive and negative reactive strategies here. It is clear we have utilised available care learning materials appropriately and it is evident that we have given in this book a good level of knowledge and understanding linked to childcare practice.

Explaining strategies used to support individuals to manage their behaviour.

As part of strategies to support positive behaviour, there are specific strategies that help individuals manage their behaviour: these strategies aim to support self-control. The individual positively works to control their challenges in behaviour. These strategies start with the concept of policy that works for a person-centred support.

- The very first thing in care that enables individuals to manage their own behaviour is communication and comprehension: the carer has to communicate, and so does the individual. Even the behaviour itself is a means of communication even if it is challenging. Messages are received by the individual from the carer, and vice versa. In order to meet the care needs of the individual effective communication must be used. The most important thing is for the carer to deal with issues that negate communication or impair it for the individual. It has been articulated that the environment, poor eyesight, lack of understanding of language or jargon and unfamiliar terms, poor or unusual use of Makaton and interpretation of sign language, hearing impairment, and speech or being non-verbal. These issues can make it difficult for communication to be effective and make it impossible for individuals to manage their own behaviour. Working with children, communication is the most effective way to care for them, and helps us to get messages across. Behaviour is learned and altered by communication, bearing in mind the lowest end of childcare is that the children are just learning everything from scratch. They learn behaviour, routine, and then giving messages; communication is the way or means of giving and receiving messages. The care that enables individuals to manage their own behaviour is the carer's recognition of various other barriers that may hinder understanding of messages being communicated to the individual intended to manage their own behaviour. Therefore carers should examine the message, examine the way it has been made, and examine if the individual has received it correctly and understood it. Carers should check if the message has been received, understood, and that there was enough time for the client to process the information/message, and/or that the appropriate method of communication is being used for the particular individual. This could be Makaton, sign language, or translation in another language. In many cases in childcare we use drawings, pictorial pictures, to get children to understand or process messages; that way we determine whether our children/clients/individuals understand messages which help them to manage their own behaviour.

- The second thing in care that enables individuals to manage their own behaviour is a carer using a system of reward strategy. There should be consistency in what is done, i.e. rewarding should mean something and the individual being able to appreciate why they are getting it, ensuring that although not all behaviour is rewarded, that it is not punishable, and carers being able to understand that whether they make rewards small or big, they are still rewards and convey the same message of goodness. Carers must ensure that others in the cared-for group see and are aware, when possible, that a reward is given for goodness. In childcare we ensure that we do not over-reward, so that we do not diminish the effect of reward and achievement for the children; so in childcare we use the "the star of the day" for the most well-behaved child of the day just before school closes. The next day all the other children aspire to manage their own behaviour so they…in the hope that…at close of school would be the star of the day. Therefore reward, such as parents rewarding with treats like a "takeaway for dinner", in care, creating a moment of going on a field trip or excursion, playing games, or even just words of praise, can all contribute to supporting individuals with their own behavioural management. Carers can help to remove the client from a situation or condition that triggers the problem behaviour, carers can communicate in a positive way, e.g. showing a choices-picture so the individual identifies what they want by pointing to what they want, enabling the individual self-help with an occupation, e.g. puzzles or iPad games, and enabling the individual to report things like bullying and abuse or marginalisation. Carers can help in training the individual to use techniques of relaxation from distress and anxiety.

- The third thing that carers can do that supports individuals to manage their own behaviour is ensuring positive approaches that are consistent and routine. This study refers to the outcome as an individual being able to apply "self-coping strategies". The consistency is to be used by the carer in dealing with any issues, but also other examples given by this course include anyone who is in direct contact with individuals, e.g. teachers;…we tell children in nursery to wash hands before and after eating, we expect parents/family to do the same; that is consistency. Other people who can help are friends, employers, colleagues, health professionals, social workers, and anyone who is helping the individual to manage their own behaviour.

- The fourth thing in care that enables individuals to manage their own behaviour is carers "establishing and dealing with the causes" of behaviour. To establish is to set up, or find. Therefore finding out the causes of behaviour enables the "dealing with, acting on" the found out behaviour. Individuals act or respond differently to the variety of likely causes of behaviour; these causes could be pain, medication, sensory issues or impairments in hearing or feeling, medical conditions or medication itself, and difficulties in conveying what need the individual has; it could be dementia or some other condition, being bullied or seeking attention, boredom or not being stimulated, anxiety, panic, and being in distress. The carer needs to establish by eliminating and identifying what it is that prompts or triggers the behaviour in order to support the individual.

Carers can find information from a "crisis prevention" website which shows the way an individual should be assisted in preventing behaviours from occurring and/or escalating and most importantly on equipping staff with skills to empower individuals to manage their own behaviour.

Care staff learn how to address disruptive behaviour; this is done through the positive behaviour management reactive strategies and the negative behaviour management strategies, and should be done safely and effectively. Once put into use the reactive strategies would increasingly support the likelihood that the individual/client will begin to choose more positive behaviours. There are six known techniques used by professional practitioners in the care that can motivate the individual's own management towards positive behaviour.

Behaviour management techniques ensure that carers use the safe and effective behaviour management strategies for remaining calm and professional during challenging situations where the individual's behaviour or triggers of behaviour that challenge are escalating.

1. Carers must be mindful of their own reaction:

It is suggested that a vital component of managing difficult behaviour is knowing that the carer's behaviour affects the behaviour of others:

- Anything the carers say or do in response to the individual's behaviour affects whether the behaviour escalates or stops.

- The carer must be aware of this factor, and when equipped and empowered with other effective and respectful behaviour management strategies, the carer then is better able to de-escalate difficult behaviour and support the individual to regain control and make positive choices.

2. Carers must maintain rational detachment from the individual/client:

- When the carer is detached in a rational manner it helps support the individual's behaviour positively in the following ways:

- The carer then maintains control.

- The carer can work and avoid the negative comments and actions from the client and not take them personally, as some may be abusive.

- The carer can maintain professionalism and not act on negatives coming from the client.

- The carer can afford to avoid instinctive reactions.

- The carer can afford not to be defensive.

A carer working and equipped with "rational detachment" can defuse escalating behaviour, as the individual sees no effect from their abuse or reactions; they wear down their challenging behaviour and encourage positive behaviour.

3. Carers have to be attentive to the needs and presence of the client/individual:

To support the management of behaviour, attention helps support positive behaviour as individuals feel valued when attended to. The carer can use facial expressions and body language to affirm the individual. Showing to the child or individual that someone is listening to them appropriately, properly, with respect. A very vital technique of care is to show the individual attention, being attentive to their call, their situation, being present with them. Individuals with or without challenging behaviour would feel:

- Unease if ignored

- On the margins of services and society, hence marginalised

- Uncared for

If an individual was upset, positive due attention can take away the anger and they begin to manage their behaviour. If individuals feel uncared for or marginalised they behave in challenging ways. It is not uncommon for individuals with behaviour that challenges to shout things like "…no one cares…"; it is at that instance the carer can shout back that "…we care…I am here…". This affirmation is supporting the individual to manage their own behaviour, through realising someone is there and they said they care.

4. Carers are trained to use positive talk:

The carer, in an effort to support the individual to manage their own behaviour, should use the self-reminder technique of "talking to oneself". The carer must reassure oneself that s/he is not the cause of the behaviour of the individual. Yet the behaviour is possibly taken out at the carer, targeting any object in sight and aiming even at the invisible. If in the heat of chaos, the carer were to think negatively such as "…I cannot deal with this…" then the plot is lost; the carer would not be able to apply all the positive and negative or reactive strategies learned. It is therefore to self-reassure, that "I can help this, I can do this…I know what and how to deal with this…" and do as trained, and call support where appropriate, but never give up on the duty of care. When individuals with challenging behaviour see that the carer is in control, they could adjust and allow themselves to be supported towards managing their own behaviour, towards positivity.

5. Carers must know their own perimeters and recognise their own limits:

Care workers have a duty to support individuals towards positive behaviour: enabling positive behaviour can come about when the individual begins to manage their own behaviour; they begin to recognise their own triggers and manage them by either calling for help or doing basics that prevent escalation of triggers into behaviour that challenges. Carers are not "jacks of all trades". A carer is a professional, but that does not make a carer someone who can deal with anything and everything. A carer who works in a team would normally have a chain of command and know that they have a supervisor or manager, and even an assistant; therefore, the carer would know who to call upon in case of support or requirement of assistance. The carer's team is for supervision, support, and assistance and backup. When a carer sees that the situation is likely to get out of control, then calling for collegial support is essential. This is part of knowing one's perimeters and limits either professionally or physically. Accept your limits and keep in mind that sometimes the best decision is to let someone else take over. In my childcare setting we sometimes have situations where very young babies need nappy changing, and in order to do so, we need one colleague to take care of the nappy whilst the other takes over looking after the other children. This way one leaves the room to change one child and another colleague takes over watching the babies that remain; one cannot do everything alone. This recognition of limits and abilities helps in enabling individuals to manage their own challenging behaviour towards positive behaviour.

6. Carers must debrief after any work session and after every serious incident:

To help the child, individual, or client to manage behaviour that challenges is good, but also good is the carer managing their own work schedule and part of that management is the good practice of debriefing. Soon after a work session or during handing over, inform the colleague taking over of what has been happening and what you have done. A carer that debriefs is one most likely to help the individual/client generate synergy to manage their own behaviour. Care is a very stressful profession; it is demanding and hard work both mentally and physically.

Therefore talking about what you, the carer, have experienced or gone through is one way to de-stress, to let it out and move on. When individuals with challenging behaviour see that the carer is in control, handing over to colleagues appropriately and debriefing, they could adjust and allow themselves to be supported towards managing their own behaviour, towards positivity.

You should have found this element of the book an excellent explanation. Take the point about a carer not being a jack of all trades, as this bluntly reflects the need for support staff to recognise the limitations of their role. From any care practice it would be arguable that consistent and positive approaches are really important when helping individuals find self-coping strategies.

How behaviour plans and support plans are used to support positive behaviour.

To describe how behaviour plans and support plans are used to support positive behaviour we very much depend on the points made through this study:

Plans are precursors, or outlines of expected action: support plans in care are documents made out for every individual to assist the carer to understand and manage the behaviour that is likely with the individual.

The behaviour support plan provides a baseline which is developed from an assessment of the individual's needs.

The baseline or foundation of a behaviour support plan is the general information taken on the admission into care of the individual.

The baseline will suggest the positive supports entitled or expected for the individual. It is the baseline/foundation support behaviour plan that ensures the nature and quality of support in order to avoid negative and poor quality care for the individual.

Carer and family observations would be taken into account when the support plan is being developed.

Behaviour specialists, e.g. clinical psychologists, engage with the family and others associated with the individual in order to develop the baseline support.

The plan becomes a guide for everyone who deals with the individual and this method equips all who care for the individual to have the same information.

The baseline support behaviour plan must be available to the carers who work with the individual, including family, friends, school or other educational facility, medical places and care homes, or respite and day-care centres. Therefore there must be a copy or access to the care plan of an individual in the places they are likely to go or be as part of maintaining consistency.

- The behaviour support plan addresses the needs of the individual and highlights the triggers likely to cause escalation and what strategies to use to support the individual towards positive behaviour.
How the support plan should look: the contents of a behaviour support plan are:

- Personal details of name, age, home address

- Details of the main carer or doctor

- Details of family/next of kin and contact

- Details of the nature and type of behaviour, frequency of occurrence of behaviour, and its level and length of time

- What causes the behaviour? E.g. debilitating aches and pains, boredom, or drawing attention

- What triggers the behaviour and which strategies work to contain it

- The plan must have proactive strategies that help support behaviour-setting guidelines, rules, routines, and boundaries so that challenging behaviour is prevented from occurring.

- The plan will include reactive strategies that help manage behaviour, used at points where the individual is becoming harmful to self or others.

- The plan will also give recovery information on support to be given following a bout of behaviour or after the situation is contained; these include reassurance or allowing calming down, examining that there are no injuries.

- The plan must show that it has been agreed upon by all those involved in the care of an individual. The individual and the family and any other professionals involved must be part of agreeing the plan.

- The plan will have in its recess a timescale for when to review it.

How to implement the behaviour support plan can be through using the strategies and making appropriate entries/records on the plan. The behaviour support plan must show the following:

1. A heading indicating the "likely situation or circumstance that can be difficult" for the individual:

These situations vary. For example it could be that the individual intends a journey, and the catching of a bus may be a problem. Has the individual been given prior notice of a journey, maybe to the doctors or to visit family?

- Where will the individual sit in the bus?

- Who is accompanying the individual?

- What happens in the bus? Is the journey short or long? Why does the bus stop at intervals (what seems like common sense may cause difficulties)? These should be recorded to ensure the plan works.

2. Displaying of behaviour that takes place. For example, when the bus stops the individual expresses aggression, when other people come in close proximity the individual may not like it and grit teeth or clench fists, flush face, speak randomly and loudly; the individual likes the bus to be moving.

3. Indication of what can be done to avoid difficult situations. For example: informing in advance that there will be a journey and it is on a bus, and that buses have other people who are also going somewhere, and the other people are not bad people. Telling the individual the bus may make many stops for different reasons such as traffic, bus stops, and traffic lights. The individual may ask questions or simply take information and accept it. When things talked about in advance occur the individual is not shocked or they do not trigger behaviour that challenges; this helps the individual to manage their own behaviour.

4. With all the best will in the world, things still happen, but when challenging behaviour occurs in, e.g. the bus situation, then the following can be done:

> When a child or individual begins to distress: It is important to engage in a conversation, or just keep talking to the individual about what is happening and where the journey is leading to. Distractions are, e.g. the videos on the telephone or iPad including a map of the journey, games, and ensuring that there is no travel anxiety.

> Should the behaviour escalate: It is recommended that the carer or accompanying worker then uses calm speech, not shouting, and the carer uses self-control of not shouting or getting angry. If self-harm is likely then it is important either to ask the bus driver to stop so the individual gets off and support/help is sought. If travel is by car it makes it easier to control the situation and to take short breaks and pacify the situation until the journey is complete.

Therefore, as shown above, plans are precursors, or provide an outline of expected action; support plans in care are documents made out for every individual to assist the carer to understand and manage the behaviour that is likely with the individual.

Monitoring the behaviour support plan:

Once the support plan for behaviour is drawn out or made, it must be shared with all the parties that work or relate and interact with the individual/client.

The care team must ensure that the behaviour support plan is effective, such that it helps the carers to manage behaviour; it helps the carers as a guide through identifying challenges, strategies, and potentials for the individual.

The plan must be researched, compiled, negotiated, and agreed upon, or if necessary amendments made and additions agreed prior to its being formally accepted and implemented by all concerned.

There must be inbuilt ways to make feedback; this course helps us to understand the tool referred to as "what's working/what's not working" to enable all carers and all who use the plan to input findings or new information in the tool.

The behaviour support plan is a working tool that can be reviewed, and such review times can be pre-scheduled within the plan, so that, e.g. after three or six months the plan is reviewed.

The support plan contains the strategies that all the carers use to interact with the individual: the carers' perspective on the strategies in the plan is very important. Therefore, as shown above, plans are precursors, or provide outlines of expected action:

The monitoring and updating of the support plans in care are documents made out for every individual to assist the carer to understand and manage the behaviour that is likely with the individual.

There are spontaneous reviews which are quick and necessary when unpredicted, unexpected, and unplanned dramatic change occurs in the behaviour or health of the individual.

You will now have got an excellent understanding of the benefits of using support plans. A carer would certainly be right to say that support plans should reflect the needs of the person and should include details of the kind of behaviour that needs to be addressed.

Explaining the importance of person-centred approaches to establishing support strategies:

Explaining the importance of person-centred approaches to establishing support strategies is to underline the description of what the care is about, i.e.:

The multi-agency approach of all who have a care responsibility for the individual, e.g. doctors, psychologist, etc. My child who suffers from Crohn's disease has a care plan where gynaecologists link with physiotherapists, the dietician, and her consultant.

The independence of the individual, allowing them to do things for themselves.

The choices of the individual, e.g. the nature of communication they choose to use, verbal, Makaton, sign, pictorial, or letter.

Rights of the individual, ensuring that the individual's rights are not violated, e.g. access to family and friends, etc.

The privacy of the individual so that there no violations, e.g. their personal and private information is secure.

Individuality, dignity, and life experience are all aspects that can be principles of person-centred approaches in planning to establish support for the individual.

Every individual has rights protected in the Human Rights Act 1998 and this has key articles that must be taken into account when care is being planned for the individual. They include:

The right to life

The prohibition of torture

The right to liberty

The freedom of thought, conscience, and beliefs

The freedom of association and prohibition of discrimination

The right to education

These rights contribute to any care plan and help carers meet the needs of the individual whilst understanding the importance of person-centred approaches to establishing support strategies.

The strategies of care are the key element in the importance of person-centred approaches to establishing support for the individual that has behaviour that challenges.

The care is to benefit the individual and any beneficial care has to deliver the following:

The individual will feel unique and valued because they are being listened to. In nursery we allow children to make their point on issues or subjects that we teach. Each gets a turn to talk.

Confidence and self-esteem are generated, as the individual experiences the importance of person-centred approaches through the established support strategies.

The individual will begin to use a wider range of skills to ensure that the quality of life is changing towards positive behaviour.

Self-support towards better behaviour may begin to happen. E.g. the individual learns self-support to prevent escalating situations.

An individual begins to take self-control of various aspects of their life, towards full human potential.

The importance of person-centred approaches to establishing support strategies will enable the individual to feel good, and they get this from being treated in ways reflecting their human rights, hence valuing them.

This book as a study enables us to understand that the importance of person-centred approaches to establishing support strategies will uphold staff awareness of the humanity of the individual and the needs they are dealing with. Skills and knowledge of staff become more effective for the individual. Families and friends get more involved, and gain confidence to care for the individual, resulting in more effective partnership with the carers. Therefore, the family, friends, and society as a whole learn that individuals receive care that is qualitative and invaluable resulting from good planning of the all-important person-centred approaches to establishing support strategies for individuals with behaviour that challenges.

This chapter now gives us an excellent explanation of person-centred approaches and the importance of such. For further information you may find the website below useful:

https://www.bapca.org.uk/about/what-is-it.html

How support networks for the individual can help promote positive behaviour:

A network is collaboration; an interconnecting, system, or grouping; therefore this is how support networks for the individual can help promote positive behaviour. These groups have to ensure they are using the same support plan.

The groups that need to be networked will include: carers, friends and family, other professionals such as psychologists, psychiatrists, neurologists, social and care workers, solicitors, advocates, mental health nurses, day-care staff, and those involved in respite care. In childcare we take on children and have to network with speech and language for speech therapists, and language development. We engage with insulin nurses and general practitioners, and in cases of special needs, we engage with social workers and the "special needs and inclusion play" teams. These groups and individuals that help the individual with challenging behaviour have to hold various meetings to discuss needs, strategy, and actions and this is how support networks for the individual can help promote positive behaviour. There are obviously diverse levels of support requirements by individuals and the networks will therefore vary accordingly.

When the support network is being developed for the individual; that target is that that network can help promote positive behaviour that challenges and bring about the promotion of positive behaviour. The network is a collaborative. That collaborative is the approach or network intended to promote positive behaviour. Where there are failings, one or more of the collaborative/network professionals has missed or not attended to the approach. The reaction from the individual is failed support. Individuals expect routine; when the nurse does not come they are stressed. In childcare where we have timetables, even at a very young age children learn to expect certain things to happen. If those things do not happen the children anxiously ask why. It is important that the network of support follows the support plan appropriately.

Whilst a network is a collaboration, an interconnecting system or grouping, and this is how support networks for the individual can help promote positive behaviour, there is a requirement on the network that there are in place "ways of monitoring and reviewing network approaches".

Training that is appropriate: training and updates on policies and procedures are critical to the success of a network and the well-being of individuals in care.

Clear and open communication lines: The network has to be in contact and regular communication of information exchange and updates to ensure that the individual is being supported through this multi-agency approach, and that each and every one is doing their expected part. There must be regular meetings of those in the network and regular conversations through letter, email, and phone.

Regular meetings of the network, particularly the key individuals: Not only the carers and professionals need to meet, but family, as well as the individual for whom care is planned, should be at meetings of those in the network and regular conversations. This way the care plan is always for the dignity of the individual. Through meetings it can be gauged what is or is not working. Through the meeting monitoring and examination of progress or lack of it is done and improvements suggested and/or included in the plan.

Ongoing monitoring: At the meetings the communication between network members helps to give an objective view of the whole person-centric approach to ensure that the plan works. This monitoring will identify gaps, if any; failings, if any; and devise solutions.

Robust reviewing of the network's actions is a way of ensuring that the plan is updated, but also bringing in best practice and looking at anything in the behaviour support plan that needs action or remedying.

This chapter is an excellent evidence of a good understanding of the learning necessary and a carer can make this material link to their own practice.

CHAPTER 7

The challenge of how the rights of clients or individuals are protected

SUMMARY OF THE LEGISLATIVE FRAMEWORK WHICH APPLIES TO CHILDREN OR INDIVIDUALS PRESENTING CHALLENGING BEHAVIOUR:

a) Rights

The legislative framework that applies to individuals who present with behaviour that challenges protects the rights of the individual:

- Human Rights Act 1998; all of health and social care is based on this act in protecting the individual.

- Equalities Act 2010; this is to ensure that the individual is protected from being discriminated or victimised on grounds of race, age, disability, gender, marital or partnership status, sex, religion, association, sexuality, or any such thing. Individuals with or without challenging behaviour have to be respected and treated with fairness and equality. Individuals have to be dealt with respectfully and ensuring their dignity without meanness. Individuals have the right to receive appropriate care and services meeting their needs without less or preferential treatment.

- Mental Capacity Act 2005 in England and Wales (Scotland 2000): This protects people over the age of sixteen who may need to have family or professionals to make all or some of the decisions on their behalf due to some incapacity. In the case of challenging behaviour the Act protects individuals to the extent that whilst some decisions may not be made by the individual due to some condition, the individual may be able to make others.

- Mental Health Act 1983 (which was amended in 2007): This is the legal application known as "being sectioned". This is the legal guidance to rights of individuals who have been diagnosed with mental illness and the law gives explicit definitions of who, how, and when an individual should be admitted to a facility, what type of treatment the individual would get, and/or if appropriate if the individual should even against their own wishes be detained in a hospital, following assessment and there is likelihood of self-harm or others.

In the first instance an interview is held to determine the well-being of the individual. Then in the second instance, as the law stipulates that no less than three professionals must concur that the individual should be sectioned under the Mental Health Act. If the individual has family, a family member would be joined by a psychiatrist, medical doctor or general practitioner, and carer who has been dealing with the individual. Some of the situations initially take place at home, a police station, or hospital as mental breakdown can occur anywhere at any time.

The Mental Health Act amendments of 2007 include:

- Expansion of professional areas when sectioning or detention of individuals could be done

- Local authority having duty of advocacy if individuals are unable to decide or speak for themselves

- The amended definition of "mental disorder"

- Appropriate medical treatment which includes new testing for individuals diagnosed with mental disorder

All these can only be effectively done in the legislative framework that applies to individuals who present with behaviour that challenges and the acts are there to protect the rights of the individual.

b) Safeguarding

To ensure comprehensive safeguarding in care, there are a number of legal acts that build up effective safeguarding:

1. The Human Rights Act 1998

2. The Equality Act 2010

3. The Mental Capacity Act 2005

4. The Mental Health Act 1983 (amended 2007)

5. The Safeguarding for Mental Capacity Act 2009

6. The Care Act 2014

7. The Safeguarding Vulnerable Groups Act 2006

Safeguarding is very important in care; it is the means by which well-being is promoted. The legislative framework that applies to individuals who present with behaviour that challenges protects the rights of the individual in this regard using the Care Act 2014. Safeguarding individuals is the duty of any local authority. Safeguarding is a major theme in care of any type. In my childcare setting safeguarding children is very important and the topmost act of caring for children, ensuring that children learn and play and are kept in a safe environment. In this course for behaviour that challenges, it is important that safeguarding is done according to the Care Act 2014:

Safeguarding therefore is evident when:

- The dignity, respect, and privacy of the individual are promoted

- Protection from abuse and neglect for the individual is upheld

- Promoting that the individual has capacity and can control care and support and their overall daily affairs

- Promoting that the individual can take part in training and work

- Promoting the welfare of domestic and family relationships

- Promoting the welfare of the individual to contribute to society and enjoy free association

The Safeguarding Vulnerable Groups Act 2006 upholds the protection of individuals so that through appropriate measures of disclosure of any criminal history, staff and carers are vetted so that those employed to work with vulnerable individuals are suitable. In my childcare setting we use a system provided through Ofsted, the watchdog for educational standards. This system links us to Disclosure and Barring Service (DBS); we are thereby able to verify if individuals have any information that excludes them from working with vulnerable people.

The individual with challenging behaviour is supported to be part of the society through care. The Care Act also ensures the safeguarding of carers or staff so that their rights are protected and welfare promoted.

c) Deprivation of liberty

The legislative framework that applies to children and individuals who present with behaviour that challenges protects the rights of the individual in this regard using the Mental Capacity Act 2009, and ensures that appropriate assessment of the individual is done to avoid:

- Administering medicine without consent unless it was legally necessary

- Being refused discharge from care facility to family or friends unless it was legally necessary

- Carers usurping all authority and decision-making unless it was legally necessary

- Being physically restrained to ensure safe admission to hospital unless it was legally necessary

To ensure safeguards against deprivation of liberty, it is imperative that there is a representative or advocate or an independent Relevant Person's Representative (RPR) for the individual if any of the above has to be done. Therefore it is only imperative that specialist trained carers can carry out particular duties to ensure safeguards from harm, abuse, or exploitation.

The above summary is giving an excellent understanding of the legislation that underpins and supports individuals who present with behaviour that challenges through disability. Should you wish to access any of the above pieces of legislation, they can be accessed at: https://www.gov.uk/

A description of the agreed ways of working to protect an individual who presents with behaviour that challenges.

This book offers a course that sets out, as seen earlier, the agreed ways of working to protect an individual who presents with behaviour that challenges, based on two principles:

1. The individual support plan

2. The set guidelines or procedures for the care of the individual

It is essential that all carers and others that work with the individual do so in a network that communicates, ensuring to use agreed strategies to enable support for the individual:

- Identify any triggers for behaviour

- Make observations objectively, identify or clarify triggers, and ensure appropriate strategies to respond to the triggers

- Positive behaviour being praised and rewarded

- Prioritise ensuring to use proactive strategies to manage behaviour before it escalates

- Take action appropriately, where proactive strategies fail, and intervene with reactive strategies

- Helping to safely support the individual with self-management of emotions and reactions

There are prescribed interventions:

The carers must always be working in agreed ways to protect an individual who presents with behaviour that challenges using appropriate prescribed interventions: as a last resort, when all else has failed to calm down the behaviour that is escalating, threatening, and becoming harmful, the interventions may be extended from instructions, verbal support to medical administration, and in cases of escalated mental disorder or behaviour deterioration to violent behaviour likely to self-harm or harm others, then intervention may take the mode of physical restraint.

Restraints take any of the following forms:

Subduing the individual's capacity to move; whole body or in part(s), e.g. arms. This is defined as "Physical Restraint".

Intervention to escort the sufferer of challenging behaviour away from a situation, or to be led away by the hand; this being "Physical Intervention".

Devices, e.g. handcuffs used to contain the individual, known as "Mechanical Restraint".

Subduing an individual through medication; this is where antipsychotic sedative substances may be medically applied and are referred to as "Chemical Restraints".

The agreed ways of working to protect an individual who presents with behaviour that challenges respects human rights; therefore in advancing human rights, there are restraints that are illegal, prohibited, and unacceptable:

It is not legal for any individual to be subjected to complete isolation.

It is not legal for any individual to be subjected to manipulation of an environment.

It is not legal for any individual to be subjected to door locks.

It is not legal for any individual to be subjected to stair gates.

Limitations of prescribed interventions:

Carers are trained to ensure that they only use appropriate and agreed ways of working to protect an individual who presents with behaviour that challenges. However, there are limitations of a prescribed intervention as follows:

Negative impact on the individual, when interventions have been applied, could include:

Decreasing of the individual's quality of life, hence poor potential.

Human rights of the individual being violated or breaches in the child(ren) or individuals' welfare.

Physical harm or injuries to the body of the child or individual: where for instance handcuffs cut into the body.

Low self-esteem can affect the individual as they feel humiliated and lose dignity, humiliating and disrespecting the individual, as the intervention may be administered without due regard to the status of the individual and their personal feelings.

Legal prescription of interventions:

Where there is likely harm to self or others, the consenting individuals would be the ideal to using restraining interventions:

To safeguard or keep safe an individual is the only instance for using restraints, which the law allows. This study makes note that failure by the carer to use restraints where an individual may injure self or others is an act of negligence. In some instances, restraints are the best option:

- When the individual consents so they feel secure and safe

- When the agreed support plan is stipulating that restraint is used to help behaviour

- When in safeguarding from self-harm or injury to self and others the restraint is applied under the Mental Act, when an individual is unable to give consent and legislation has been adhered to

The above explains the agreed ways of working to protect an individual who presents with behaviour that challenges and these ways uphold and respect human rights. This is an excellent explanation. It is clear that you will now have recognised that interventions could include:

- Physical

- Mechanical

- Chemical

The above explanation motivates a good use of learning, giving material and evidence applicable from, e.g. a childcare experience and practice.

Describing how to monitor interventions and safeguard individuals.

In describing how to monitor interventions and safeguard individuals we must take account of the facts that:

1. Monitoring is to remind, caution, or admonish; so that we ensure correct action of care because we are cautious.

2. Interventions are the actions intended to bring about the desired support for behavioural needs.

3. Safeguarding is the ensuring that those receiving any type of care are safe, in a safe environment, and their dignity not violated, that they are free from abuse or harm and exploitation.

4. Who the individual is: the individual is the one receiving care and has human rights and liberties that must be respected.

The continued or ongoing use of interventions has to be monitored to ensure that individuals are safeguarded in the light of human rights preservation and sustenance. The care industry monitors the strategies of intervention, recording them and reviewing them, then those strategies that seem defective or detrimental to human rights are revoked and new ones or updates are put in place. The keeping of records is the basis for reviewing of strategies.

- Good record-keeping is part and parcel of the policies in place in any care setting.

- How records are managed is important for the treatment and welfare of clients and the competence and safety of staff.

- Records help in the monitoring of interventions to ensure the safeguarding of individuals in care and they are useful:

- For adequate and relevant care to be in place, records are kept as a point of reference; all carers for the individual would have access to such records in order to carry out appropriate service to meet the needs of that individual.

- The records are used when new strategies are being developed and any irrelevant or out-of-date strategies scrapped. In some instances, restraints are the best option:

- Records help in ensuring the use of current strategies for the individual.

- Records contain information on prescribed interventions, which may include restraints, therefore the monitoring of the records is important to ensure the correct action is taken.

- Records show reasons or grounds for the use of restraints, the justification or rationale for the use of particular restraints.

- Records contain the original observation and discussions including the overall consenting and legal justification for the use of restraints on an individual.

- Records also detail objective observations and preferred strategies for the use of restraints.

- The records will also hold any injuries that are either historical or resulting from use of past application of restraints and what action was taken to alleviate injuries or treat them.

- Details of time and day or dates when restraints were used, or necessary, and the nature of restraints are kept on record.

- The records ensure that the monitoring of interventions and safeguarding individuals is kept current to ensure the support plan and baseline services are in line with the supporting of the needs of the individual.

- The keeping of records can ensure that the human rights of the client are protected through monitoring of interventions and safeguarding individuals in care.

- The safety of the individual is upheld when the records are kept and monitored.

- Record-keeping helps maintain accuracy of actions and strategies to support behaviour; therefore, the monitoring of interventions and safeguarding individuals, when kept current, helps carers ensure the support plan and baseline services so that they are in line with the supporting of the needs of the individual.

In the care services we must avoid poor record-keeping:

The consequences of poor record-keeping are grave: poor record-keeping or the failure to keep records is due to poor training and management:

Where there are no records, incidents are not recorded and acted upon appropriately; care for individuals becomes questionable.

With poor record-keeping or in the absence of records, staff do not have awareness of restraints, their nature, use, or what generally constitutes them.

Without appropriate record-keeping the rights of individuals are easily floundered.

Where there is no record-keeping, guidelines are not in place and there is a lack of points of reference to use correct strategies.

Therefore, record-keeping helps the monitoring of interventions and safeguarding individuals, in order to keep abreast with the current information on the care support plan and baseline services that are necessary for supporting of the needs of the individual.

In describing how to monitor interventions and safeguard individuals we must take account of the facts that:

1. Monitoring is to remind, caution, or admonish; so that we ensure correct action of care because we are cautious.

2. Interventions are the actions intended to bring about the desired support for behavioural needs.

3. Safeguarding is the ensuring that those receiving any type of care are safe, in a safe environment, and their dignity not violated, that they are free from abuse or harm and exploitation.

4. Who the individual is: the individual is the one receiving care and has human rights and liberties that must be respected.

The continued or ongoing use of interventions has to be monitored to ensure that individuals are safeguarded in the light of human rights preservation and sustenance. The care industry monitors the strategies of intervention, recording them and reviewing them, then those strategies that seem defective or detrimental to human rights are revoked and new ones or updates are put in place. The keeping of records is the basis for reviewing of strategies.

- Good record-keeping is part and parcel of the policies in place in any care setting.

- How records are managed is important for the treatment and welfare of clients and the competence and safety of staff.

- Records help in the monitoring of interventions to ensure the safeguarding of individuals in care and they are useful:

- For adequate and relevant care to be in place, records are kept as a point of reference; all carers for the individual would have access to such records in order to carry out appropriate service to meet the needs of that individual.

- The records are used when new strategies are being developed and any irrelevant or out-of-date strategies scrapped.

- Records help in ensuring the use of current strategies for the individual.

- Records contain information on prescribed interventions, which may include restraints, therefore the monitoring of the records is important to ensure the correct action is taken.

- Records show reasons or grounds for the use of restraints, the justification or rationale for the use of particular restraints.

- Records contain the original observation and discussions including the overall consenting and legal justification for the use of restraints on an individual.

- Records also detail objective observations and preferred strategies for the use of restraints.

- The records will also hold any injuries that are either historical or resulting from use of past application of restraints and what action was taken to alleviate injuries or treat them.

- Details of time and day or dates when restraints were used, or necessary, and the nature of restraints are kept on record.

- The records ensure that the monitoring of interventions and safeguarding individuals is kept current to ensure the support plan and baseline services are in line with the supporting of the needs of the individual.

- The keeping of records ensures that the human rights of the client are protected through monitoring of interventions and safeguarding individuals in care.

- The safety of the individual is upheld when the records are kept and monitored.

- Record-keeping helps maintain accuracy of actions and strategies to support behaviour; therefore, the monitoring of interventions and safeguarding individuals, when kept current, helps carers ensure the support plan and baseline services so that they are in line with the supporting of the needs of the individual.

In the care industry we must avoid poor record-keeping:

The consequences of poor record-keeping are grave. Poor record-keeping or the failure to keep records is due to poor training and management:

Where there are no records, incidents are not recorded and acted upon appropriately; care for individuals becomes questionable.

With poor record-keeping or in the absence of records, staff don't have awareness of restraints, their nature, use, or what generally constitutes them.

Without appropriate record-keeping the rights of individuals are easily floundered.

Where there is no record-keeping, guidelines are not in place and there is a lack of points of reference to use correct strategies.

Therefore, record-keeping helps the monitoring of interventions and safeguarding individuals, in order to keep abreast with the current information on the care support plan and baseline services that are necessary for supporting the needs of the individual.

Within the above information you are shown how to reflect the importance of good record-keeping. It is important to document any incidents of behaviour that challenges, any triggers to this situation, what interventions were used, and how effective they were.

CHAPTER 8

The challenge of understanding the importance of effective communication and the management of challenging behaviour

COMMUNICATION IN MANAGING BEHAVIOUR

The identified range of communication methods includes the following:

Verbal, the spoken or said word; where the individual talks.

Non-verbal; where the individual may not talk, speak, or say words, but use gestures or movements and indications of body.

Written; this being the writing in any style or language of expressions that could otherwise have been said or spoken.

Pictorials; when pictures or drawings are used to convey the message that would have otherwise been said or spoken.

Makaton, Sign; this is sign language by the hands or fingers.

Technological communication; using equipment to generate messages and conveying them, e.g. telephones, iPads.

The above identified range of communication is a means of human interaction to uphold or enhance individual potential in understanding one another: in the case of behaviour that challenges, communication is the all-important factor that enables carers to care and support behaviour so that it does not escalate to harmful levels for the individual or others around the individual. Relationships that are positive are founded and built upon effective communication. The task for the carer is to ensure that appropriate interpretation is made of any type of communication made by the individual. The carer has a duty to identify the preferred method of communication for the individual in care, which usually should be on the support plan. The benefits of communication for the individual with behavioural challenge will include the following:

- Giving information, about themselves or their needs

- Identifying and finding out information about their behaviour, etc.

- Convey or express their feelings, i.e. emotional status

- Ensuring that their needs are known, to enable carers to meet them

- Help interact to make friendships or developing relationships

- Observe and cope with social norms

- Enabling other people to accept the individual's position, i.e. persuasion

The identified range of communication methods shows that communication is expression:

Communication shows that individuals use behaviour as a form of expression: identifying a range of communication methods clearly shows how behaviour is a form of expression: individuals with challenging behaviour do so resulting from a variety of issues and information may need to be communicated to them in particular ways. They too find expressions the alternative to something they cannot verbalise: my child with autism used to just run away from situations that she found unpleasant; if, e.g. we are walking on the pavement and an ambulance or police siren was sounded from a vehicle, or if a loud motorbike went past. We later realised after professional diagnosis that she also had sensory issues of sound and smell. Therefore, through behaviour many individuals with challenging behaviour are actually trying to express or communicate messages that carers should not overlook, but interpret carefully.

The identified range of communication methods also shows that common behaviour means something: the carer has a duty to verify if the behaviour is associated with isolation, loneliness, anger, fear, medication, need for fresh air, toilet, or is it pain and discomfort? The carer monitoring the behaviour would also get information from the support plan, to know what strategies to apply for the individual when that individual makes particular expressions in behaviour.

Supporting individuals using the identified range of communication methods includes the specialist attention for the individuals who use only non-verbal communication: the individual is intelligent but has no vocal ability and would benefit from other methods of communication. In cases of non-verbal communication, facial expressions, gesturing, body posturing, and proximity are means of effective communication with individuals or clients. There are many non-verbal individuals who are able to write; this method then enables them to use written communication. If the individual prefers written communication to gestures or sign language, the support plan should clearly set that out for carers to use.

AAC, the Augmentative and Alternative Communication Method: As we discuss the identified range of communication methods carers must understand that there are a variety of means that help communication including the following:

1. Symbols: They give clear and quick information and they help challenging behaviour. Symbols in the day-to-day situation are used for drivers or road users to avoid accidents.

2. Objects: the clear message of objects such as showing the individual a teacup or a fork, etc. helps reinforce messages and makes communication.

3. Photos/diagrams: the photos and diagrams can enable an individual to communicate and/or understand messages.

Therefore, the identified range of communication methods are very instrumental in care, such that individuals receiving care are understood, and that carers can communicate effectively. The identified range of communication methods includes the discovery of new and cultural methods devised to enable individuals to receive good care. Such a method is:

MAKATON and BRITISH SIGN LANGUAGE (BSL): There is distinction between Makaton and BSL, and due to the complex nature of BSL Makaton is usually preferred by users of sign language. Sign language uses hands, facial, and body expressions. Makaton is symbolic and users find it simpler than BSL. It is important that carers can distinguish which method is being used by the individual with behavioural challenges.

The identified range of communication methods includes PECS; this is "The Picture Exchange Communication System". These can be made available for carers to use with the individual with challenging behaviour.

PECS supports the communication of the individual and can enhance interaction with carers and others improving the quality of life for the individual.

Human aids are among the identified range of communication methods: human aids are people who convey messages, they are go-betweens, they bridge the space between the individual with needs and the carer in instances where communication is needed but not being achieved. These could include interpreters or translators of language, but even more complex, the go-between can be an advocate who speaks or writes with authority for and on behalf of the individual.

The identified technological range of communication methods includes the following: hearing aids to support poor hearing reception, reinforcing the ability to hear and improve the quality of life. Carers must be observant and should always find information on the support plan to make sure if the hearing aid is used and actually switched on or regularly serviced to work effectively. There is now new technological communication such as iPads and mobile telephones, where messages can be sent verbally or in text-written form. Carers can ensure that the individual is comfortable and competent in the use of mobile telephone or iPad so that care is effective. Also in the identified technological range of communication methods is included VOCAs, the "Voice Boxes or Voice Output" communication aids: these store voice messages, which are then replayed to the individual as appropriate. Because these operate by touchscreen or button, they help in physiotherapy especially for body movements. Babies benefit in the use of similar implements where they can listen to familiar voices, e.g. of their parent, and this enables carers to support behaviour positively.

The above information gives an excellent depiction which correctly identified a range of communication methods including:

- Verbal communication

- Non-verbal communication

- Written communication

- Use of pictures

- Technology

The importance of non-verbal communication

The importance of non-verbal communication is that it constitutes the majority of the interactive message conveyance between people; estimates are that 50% to 80% non-verbal communication takes place between people in any exchange. There are various ways of non-verbal communication including the following:

- Expressions of the face: This is extremely important as it becomes the first impression of meeting or communicating with others; facial expressions can either be welcoming or forbidding. This helps in care as individuals receiving care can make facial expressions to convey their needs to carers.

- Posture of the body: This also conveys expressions to others; either we are interested by leaning forward towards the individual or folding our hands defensively, or disinterested, or again with open arms we are welcoming. This helps in care as individuals receiving care can enable carers to interpret the body posture of an individual to apply appropriate strategies.

- Gesticulation: This is making gestures, and is very common in day-to-day communication. Individuals nod in agreement and shake heads from side to side to indicate disagreement. This helps in care as individuals receiving care can make gestures indicating what their need is.

- Approximation: This is proximity, the act of being close or drawing together; the closeness with which an individual gets to another person indicates information. When individuals move away from another either they have finished working/interacting with them, they are uninterested, or have other things to tend to. However, proximity is communication, which can be indicating goodness or even threatening.

Non-verbal communication and cultural norms:

Culture or the environment in which people are is very important when delivering care: culture dictates the expressions and verbal communication that people use; what messages and how those messages are received is very important in care work. There are cultures where whistling is taken as offensive. There are others where particular signage or symbols would be acceptable and others unacceptable. Therefore carers for individuals with behaviour that challenges need to ensure that the sign or symbols they would use are appropriate and would not be misconstrued. Where non-verbal communication is used the carer must ensure that the client will understand and that support for behaviour would be positive.

Effects of specific conditions on communication:

The identified range of communication methods may be affected by particular or specific conditions that bear on the individual: the effects to communication, e.g. where symbols are used and the individual has impaired vision, may not have the desired effect or the full benefit of seeing the symbols. Therefore there are six specific aspects that can affect communication, namely:

- Dementia: This mainly occurs with old age and can cause a range of communication problems including short span memory, long-term memory, failure to recognise people or things, concentration or focus, understanding messages or issues, and loss of perception. This sort of situation causes difficulties and can affect behaviour.

- ADHD: Attention Deficit Hyperactivity Disorder

- Learning differences

- Down's syndrome

- Mental disability/mental health conditions

- Physical disability/physical restrictions

- Sensory impairments/issues

Therefore, specific health or even environmental conditions can affect communication for individuals, and carers need to ensure appropriate support.

In view of specific conditions dictating effects of communication: the individual/client could communicate needs in different ways:

Through observations during care and prior to implementing the support plan the carers have the opportunity to make assessments and analyses to make conclusions on how the client may be communicating their needs through behaviour: the question for the carer is "What is the individual trying to communicate?" This observation has enabled the care industry to surmise that some traits although from different individuals usually convey a similar message. For instance: an individual may show signs of behaving "restlessly not being able to focus or settle". In this instance the client may be in pain, or irritated, or need to go to the toilet, etc. This course also teaches us that "shouting" is a common behaviour of communicating that the individual is either feeling ignored, unattended to, or isolated. It has been suggested that overstimulation of the individual by environmental surroundings, e.g. hot or cold environment, can cause shouting. The individual with behaviour that challenges could exhibit "repetitive and ritualistic" mannerisms which convey messages of anxiety, dislike of the current environment, boredom, or to try to draw attention to them.

To support positive behaviour through communication, therefore, carers must know that specific health or even environmental conditions can affect communication for individuals, and carers need to ensure appropriate support.

This chapter has so far given an excellent picture of what a carer needs to know and correctly identified a range of communication methods including:

- Verbal communication

- Non-verbal communication

- Written communication

- Use of pictures

- Technology

CHAPTER 9

The challenge of describing barriers to communication

ADDRESSING BARRIERS TO COMMUNICATION:

Communication means interaction, whilst barriers refer to hindrances. For carers to clearly describe barriers to communication is to understand that "barriers to communication are a main cause" of behavioural challenges in individuals. There are three potential ways of barriers; namely, the message communicated is not received, understanding the message has been distorted, message communication is received but that message is not or is misunderstood. Individuals with challenging behavioural issues may exhibit or experience all three ways or some of these hindrances to effective communication.

The three barriers should be understood as follows:

- Communication is received but that message is not or is misunderstood: this is when an individual/client has psychological or mental issues; there are barriers to understanding particular things unless communicated in a particular manner.

- Message communicated is not received: this is in many instances, when for instance someone has a hearing impediment, or visual problems, or language is not familiar, even signed language not understood, or they cannot see the signing.

- Understanding the message has been distorted: This is where for instance translators or interpreters are not familiar with a language dialect or cultural usage, and for individuals with challenging behaviour, it may be that they do not understand due to any number of factors associated with a disability, etc. Therefore the carer has a task to ensure that any hindrance to communication is managed to ensure the support towards positive behaviour.

There are examples of hindrances to communication which include:

1. The surrounding, or local environment: Complex health needs may cause an individual to feel uncomfortable; discomfiture causes complications, and if someone is in a care environment, they may feel restricted or develop a dislike to such an environment. Many times a room may cause difficulties for an individual resulting in the environment becoming a barrier to communication.

2. Making assumptions about the individual: The problems of failure in care arise when assumptions are made about the client. Even if you think you know how they behave or react do not make assumptions; analyse, observe, and respond positively to communication, otherwise

assumptions can become a barrier to communicating with the individual and fail positive behavioural management.

3. Technical language/dialects/slang/accents: The daily language used may be for instance English, but if English is spoken by someone who uses other languages or slang or dialects, the client, who may be from a different background, may not understand immediately what is being communicated. Carers need to become aware of these issues and communicate as clearly and slowly as possible, asking the individual if they have understood so that slang or technical language does not become a barrier to communication.

4. Sensory issues or sensory impairments: The barrier in communication is created by not seeing, not hearing, not smelling, and not feeling. For the individual with sensory issues, they may not get communication messages purely because they could not see or hear. The carer must make an all-round assessment and observe if the individual has sensory issues that need tending to or else the communication will be hindered.

5. Drugs and/or alcohol can hinder communication: There is always a barrier that develops from excessive intoxicant consumption such as alcohol or drug use. When behaviour that challenges combines with intoxicants the situation becomes escalated and communication in most such cases will be hindered. Carers may have to detox or allow time for the individual to regain sobriety to communicate with them effectively.

6. Language needs and preferences: The individual with challenging behaviour will normally like to communicate in a manner that they are used to. Anxiety and weariness can develop if the individual is not allowed to communicate in a language they prefer or know well. Language can be a barrier if not understood. All effort has to be made at the outset that individuals with challenging behaviour understand and are understood, to work towards positive behaviour.

7. Mental illness: When people are diagnosed with schizophrenia and other mental illnesses usually the communication is hindered. Some people with acute or severe depression find barriers in speech or understanding messages. It is important that carers will comprehend these barriers in order to work well with individuals that need care.

8. Cultural differences: the cultural differences or varieties of the global village are immense; there is a need to understand the cultural environment that the carer works in so that communication finds no barriers; the use of slogans or words that are unfamiliar to individuals will create difficult barriers and communication would be hindered.

9. Personality privacy/confidentiality: Here the carer has to tease information from the individual that needs care, especially at the initial observation or analyses before a support plan is devised; personality differs from individual to individual. There are individuals who feel their health information is private and cannot be shared and will hesitate in making any disclosure. This personality trait will become a barrier to communication if the individual withholds information about themselves.

Therefore the carer has a task to ensure that any hindrance to communication is managed to ensure the support towards positive behaviour. The carer has a duty to overcome the barriers to enhance the communication between carer and client/individual especially in situations of challenging behaviour.

Significant aspects in overcoming communication barriers:

Communication helps the carer convey the message that they are there to support the individual. The individual with need is only able to convey their need through communication whether verbal, non-verbal, or behavioural. The reasons for overcoming communication hindrances include:

- Reducing negative feelings and emotions: it is important to create a situation of safety and security for the individual so they have trust and confidence in order to communicate their needs, but also support positive behavioural outcomes.

- De-escalating the circumstances: it is important that the situation that may have escalated should be managed, but to do so effectively communication has to take place with the carer implementing the strategies to deal with the triggers and ensure that calmness is restored to support positive behaviour.

- Appropriate understanding of the client: it is important that when there is better understanding of the individual, the communication hindrance is removed, because the carer gets to know what the needs are as the individual communicates them and as the carer communicates appropriate support towards positive behaviour.

- Understanding and using tools of communication: It is important that carers must increase their own awareness of tools of communication with individuals and the variety of needs and cultures. The carer must draw from the availability of tools, such as their knowledge, equipment, and colleague support, to remove communication barriers and support behaviour.

- Increasing self-confidence and esteem: it is important that carers acknowledge the importance of increased self-esteem where the individual's ability to socialise and interact with others improves communication and takes away barriers that would otherwise hinder communication.

- Reducing any misunderstandings: It is important that carers remove situations of misunderstanding in communication. This is where clear routines and timetables help so that the individual receiving care understands and knows what to expect, to support positive behaviour.

Therefore in this course we learn that the carer has a task to ensure that any hindrance to communication is managed to ensure the support towards positive behaviour. The carer has a duty to overcome the barriers to enhance the communication between carer and client/individual especially in situations of challenging behaviour.

The significance of awareness of own behaviour to deal with barriers of communication:

Awareness of your own behaviour as a carer is very important when dealing with barriers to communication in situations of challenging behaviour. The task for the carer is never to take things simply at face value, because there may be underlying issues triggering the behaviour of an individual.

The questions to ask as a carer are:

Who am I? What am I to do here? Do I understand my role? And how shall I conduct myself when the behaviour of the client escalates?

The answers to these simple questions would help the carer not to be flippant in the situation. And in order to be vigilant the carer would have five points in mind:

1. Not to have poor attitude or behaviour towards the client or individual who needs care. The client must be respected in order that the needs are addressed; therefore the carer should ensure good and vigilant attitude and manners. Ensuring awareness of own behaviour as a carer is as good a carer by the way they respond to barriers of communication.

2. Carers must not have poor awareness of the complexities of the individual's needs: This is important as it impacts on the behaviour of the carer to respond with the correct attitude and manners to the needs of the individual ensuring that the treatment given is equal to that of any other individual in the same condition. Therefore the carer should ensure good and vigilant attitude and manners, ensuring awareness of own behaviour as a carer, as it is good to respond to barriers of communication.

3. Carers must never be unaware that they have provided insufficient information: Clients require adequate information, and in the bustle of care it is important that carers should be aware that information provided is likely to be inadequate for the individual, e.g. on the use of medication, therefore the carer should not hesitate to repeat instructions and information and ask whether the individual has any questions to ensure that information is communicated adequately. Therefore the carer should ensure good and vigilant attitude and manners; ensuring awareness of own behaviour as a carer in order to respond to barriers of communication.

4. Carers must not abuse their powers: There are situations where carers could take matters into their hands so to say, i.e. making decisions for individuals in care without due consultation. This is wrong and can be classed as abuse of responsibility and authority. The carer is there to help the individual support their own behaviour towards self-esteem and be in control of their own behaviour and overall life. Carers providing care should never get annoyed and act with anger, but always with self-control; thereby the carer should ensure good and vigilant attitude and manners, ensuring awareness of their own behaviour as a carer to be able to respond to barriers of communication.

5. Carers must never have different values and beliefs to an individual: Individuals can make requests and statements. In situations where a carer is asked by the client/individual in care for something that is not in line or values of the carer, the carer should be sensitive to the needs of the   individual.
Self-awareness of the carers ensures good and vigilant attitudes and manners, ensuring awareness of own behaviour as a carer which is good to respond to barriers of communication. When a carer is self-aware it would enable them to implement the variety of "ways to overcome barriers to communication".

The above information is an excellent provision of an array of examples of barriers to communication. Other examples can be found by accessing the following website: https://www.skillsyouneed.com/ips/barriers-communication.html

The ways or methods to overcome barriers to communication

<u>**The various ways to overcome communication barriers:**</u>

In a talk on communication, for relations, given by one called Cutlip in 1952, he identified the seven C's that help overcome barriers. These included:

1. Clarity: ensuring that communication is clear without ambiguity.

2. Credibility: carer must communicate well, be credible, and their work of quality.

3. Content: the content of communication must be valid.

4. Context: the context of communication must be correct and appropriate to be valued.

5. Continuity: there must be flow and continuity to communication for it to bear meaning.

6. Capability: the communication must be capable of conveying the intended message.

7. Channels: there must be channels of communication, e.g., verbal, translation, Makaton (Source: https://www.educba.com).

There are generally seven C's in every aspect of human communication which help in overcoming any barriers that can be brought about by individuality, personal or social circumstances, or environment.

Through this study we learn that: overcoming any type of barrier takes into account their nature, the individual, and the carer. It is essential to implement the care method set out in the support plan to respond to barriers of communication. This study enables us to learn that there are several ways to overcome communication barriers and sets out the following examples:

- Build a relationship helping the individual to feel valued and respected so that they respond positively to communication to manage or control their own behaviour using the person-centred approach.

- Carers should maintain appropriate attitudes, using self-reflection and taking on the task of ensuring safety and care when dealing with clients/individuals such that all the training they got kicks in showing that they are interested in the client, not displaying ignorance or any arrogance. This way the barriers to communication will be overcome.

- Carer-staff training: Training does help improve skills in any profession to fill the gaps of service delivery; enriching knowledge in care. That way, transmissions of knowledge, e.g. about mental illness, culture, and various means of communication or new tools are learned to improve communication and reduce barriers ensuring that the carer can support to de-escalate behaviour for individuals.

- Carers must meet self-esteem needs: When in need of care most people become dependent, and vulnerability comes with need. Carers can overcome communication barriers by creating rapport with the client, show clients they are valued, making them feel safe and respected, in order to build self-esteem; showing the carers are interested in the client and are ready to support or assist.

- Carers need to observe behaviour and identify any signs of triggers: Good practice by carers will enable them to carry out the task of care which is to continually evaluate the needs of the individual and this can only be done effectively by observations of how the client is behaving and identifying any likely causes or triggers. If carers are observant, they communicate with the client/individual and are in position to defuse challenging situations competently.

- Adapting use of a preferred method or way of communication helps overcome communication barriers because for instance if it is language, get in an interpreter or translator; PECS and Makaton could be drawn in to support the individual's needs, so that the barrier of communication is removed.

- Carers can use "active listening"; clearly showing the individual that s/he is being listened to will remove communication barriers. This can be reinforced by not interrupting them when they are talking or communicating by any other means but wait and listen and then interact when they pause. If interrupted, individuals feel ignored and undermined.

- Carers can make changes to the environment where the care is being done, to enable good temperature, lighting, and noise levels or change the location of care, e.g. a room to another room. Environment plays a big part in removing communication barriers and particularly with individuals that have challenging behaviour.

When a carer is self-aware it would enable them to implement the variety of "ways to overcome barriers to communication".

Examples of how communication can be adapted to meet the needs and preferences of each individual.

Examples of how communication can be adapted to meet the needs and preferences of each individual are many and varied:

1. These examples are the alternative methods of communication: these examples help to remove barriers of understanding between carer and client. These examples enable the removal of difficulty in communication.

- AAC: the augmentative and alternative communication, which is a complement to verbal or spoken words, AAC uses pictorial/photos and symbols and is an example of how communication can be adapted to meet the needs and preferences of each individual.

- Makaton and Sign language, which in Britain is referred to as BSL, adapted for enabling communication for those suffering hearing impediments. Makaton is simplified sign language and serves the same communication aims.

- Technical aids, such as iPads, phones, and hearing aids, can help remove communication barriers thereby providing alternative examples of adapted means to meet the needs of the individual. In childcare we find children fascinated by the same subject matter especially when it involves an iPad than when it is not.

- PECS (Picture Exchange Communication System); this is an example wherein the clients are assisted to use photos from their saved album and are able to identify what they wish to convey using the photo or picture. The PECS use is an alternative way that helps enhance the communication and interaction between client and carer.

- Translation/interpretation is another alternative showing how communication can be adapted to meet the needs and preferences of each individual. Translation and/or interpretation helps individuals understand what carers are saying and carers are able to understand what individuals/clients are saying.

2. Using the general rules of communication also shows how communication can be adapted to meet the needs and preferences of each individual. The effort is to make effective communication, effective messaging, and effective understanding. The guidelines that help make effective the alternative methods are as follows:

- Carers should simplify matters, and not use unnecessary jargon or complicated technical terms, so that the client can interact and communicate effectively, and this is how communication can be adapted to meet the needs and preferences of each individual.

- Carers should be sensitive, through observation and monitoring; ensuring that the client is actually understanding. There is no harm in repeating something twice or saying it a different way, showing an example of it or a picture where uncertainty of comprehension is detected. This is how communication can be adapted to meet the needs and preferences of each individual.

- Carers should use the alternative communication when clients are alert and not drowsy, e.g. from medication.

- Carers must allow interaction, so that conversation is uninterrupted especially when the client is communicating; therefore plenty of time must be allowed to listen and hear out the client.

- Carers must ensure that in the use of alternative communication, the situation, location, and overall environment is conducive, without unnecessary bright or flash lighting, no unwanted background noise interruptions, etc. That environment contributes to how communication can be adapted to meet the needs and preferences of each individual.

- Carers must use clarity of language, body language, or posture and sustain eye contact when using alternative means of communication. However there are cultural differences that should be taken account of, yet this is how communication can be adapted to meet the needs and preferences of each individual.

- The carer must be patient and ensure active and sustained listening to the communication of a client. It is not appropriate to interrupt the client; allow time and patiently listen, then respond when the client has finished saying their bit. This is how communication can be adapted to meet the needs and preferences of each individual.

Therefore as shown above general rules for conversation are an example of how communication can be adapted to meet the needs and preferences of each individual.

3. Carers using the "person-centred approach in care" also show how communication can be adapted to meet the needs and preferences of each individual. To use person-centred approaches will enable positive behaviour; challenges would be de-escalated and communication enhanced. The person-centred approaches include:

i). Carers being "consistent" in communicating. Because any communication with inconsistencies will convey confusing messages that can create anxiety and escalation of behaviour. All those who support the individual, e.g. family, friends, professionals, and the carers must ensure consistency in communication.

ii). Carers must ensure that the approaches used are personalised or person-centred: This way communication will target and meet all the needs, whilst in their preferred language the decisions are made by the client, the carer is ensuring that communication is flowing effectively. This is how communication can be adapted to meet the needs and preferences of each individual.

iii). Carers must uphold "age-appropriate" communication, so that the self-esteem of individuals is upheld, not speaking with adults as if they were children; due respect must be accorded to clients; their vulnerability is a result of need and must not be used to humiliate them. This approach shows how communication can be adapted to meet the needs and preferences of each individual.

4. Interpretation/translation no-go areas: Alternative approaches of communication are a positive way of carers promoting how communication can be adapted to meet the needs and preferences of each individual. However carers should not use children or family members to interpret or translate:

- Family members could be distressed or agitated with what is being conveyed.

- A child may misunderstand what is being asked of them to interpret.

- Family members could be very emotionally charged; the child being asked to translate could fail to suppress their own emotions.

- Family members may fail to grasp the technical messages in the communication. It is important therefore to get professional translators or interpreters to assist in the situation and that is how communication can be adapted to meet the needs and preferences of each individual.

This chapter has therefore made an excellent use of examples here of how communication can be adapted to meet the needs and preferences of each child or individual being cared for. It is evident in the above section that the approach is very person-centred—this is an essential quality to have in the caring profession. This concept was introduced by Carl Rogers—for further information please find below a useful website, should you wish to conduct any further reading:

https://www.bapca.org.uk/about/what-is-it.html

The challenge to explain the impact or effects that communication can make on others.

The effects that communication can have on others in a care environment are immense: carers impact the life of an individual through communication, whether that communication is body language, i.e. gesture or a smile, or verbal, i.e. something spoken or said. If communication is poorly harnessed towards a client, the following negative effects could occur:

- Escalation of challenging behavioural incidents

- Failure of meeting the needs or resolving problems

- Loneliness or isolation and marginalisation

- Loss of confidence, destruction of trust in carers

- Loss of esteem and feeling humiliated

The above negative effects occur in the behaviour of individuals who have challenging behaviour when communication is poorly harnessed towards them. To avoid these negative consequences the care worker should exercise self-awareness. The care worker should use the care skill of subconsciously asking oneself:

- Who am I?

- How am I?

- What am I doing and what am I here to do?

- What's required of me?

- What am I saying?

- What body language am I displaying?

- What effect is all this having on my client?

- What am I saying verbally?

- What am I expressing in my face, my words, gestures?

These self-examination questions will enhance oneself-awareness of the carer and enhance the response and positive actions intended to support communication when caring for individuals with behaviour that challenges.

The significance of self-awareness:

All professional care should use the care skill of subconsciously using self-awareness during interaction with individuals, so that the care worker is then not a trigger for escalation of behaviour, but a support towards positive behaviour. Staff or carers must reflect on behaviour or expressions whenever they encounter that in their presence an individual's behaviour escalates with agitation and challenges. This could be caused by verbal, non-verbal communication. This study suggests reflection on carers:

~ Showing interest in the individual, eye contact, listen attentively and actively

~ Vocal volume; is it too loud when they speak or too low that the individual can't hear?

~ Does the carer stand too far away or come too close in proximity to the individual?

~ What facial expressions are used? When are the expressions used? Are they facial or gestures?

~ Is the carer using the client's preferred communication method or not?

~ The carer must always avoid gestures that infuriate the client/individual with behaviour that challenges, e.g. pointing fingers at them.

~ The carer should not interrupt individuals but must listen and then interact.

~ As a carer you must allow time, so individual can respond to any verbal or gesture communication; self-awareness will enable carers to ensure that they do not do something whilst trying at the same time to communicate with the individual.

Through self-awareness carers become more focussed and robust in mannerism and methodology, using strategies appropriately. To increase self-awareness:

- A carer can increase self-awareness by noting down best examples of practice.

- A carer can increase self-awareness by sharing with colleagues and implementing experiences of best practice.

- A carer can increase self-awareness by seeking comments from colleagues after observing what that carer does.

- A carer can increase self-awareness by going on courses that focus on self-awareness.

- A carer can increase self-awareness by letting other people observe their work and then examining their reactions, then making adjustments as recommended.

Therefore, through self-awareness carers become more focussed and robust in mannerism and methodology, using strategies appropriately.

CHAPTER 10

The challenge of how to manage challenging behaviour

MANAGEMENT OF BEHAVIOUR:

Explaining the importance of positive reinforcement.

In psychology the importance of positive reinforcement is that it aims to use modification of reward strategies to ensure that the individual is supported to achieve positive behaviour: the importance of positive reinforcement can encourage individuals to continue towards positive behaviour. The reward or reinforcement is most effective when the positive behaviour occurs and the reward is given; then the individual is most likely to remember why the reward was given.

The importance of positive reinforcement is seen through four clear methods:

1. The Natural Reinforcements: This study gives the instance of how the number of friends and groups of people who can visit or interact with the individual can be increased when more positive behaviour is shown. The better the behaviour, the more opportunities to interact with other or new people.

2. The Token Reinforcements: This reinforcement is one such example that works very well with children who have, e.g. autism. They get a sticker as a token of good behaviour and this can continue whenever good behaviour happens.

3. The Social Reinforcers: Praising individuals when they do well is an example of reinforcing good behaviour; this way whenever the individual interacts well with others a shout of "Well done! Well done!" echoes out. This positive reinforcement then activates positive behaviour.

4. The Tangible Reinforcements: something to hold on to as an achievement is a positive reinforcement when given as a reward for good action, and for individuals with challenging behaviour, this enables and enhances supported positive behaviour.

The usefulness of positive reinforcement:

Reinforcements give strength to behaviour; so the process to achieve positive behaviour is the "positive reinforcements". The importance of positive reinforcement is that it provides the carer with one of the powerful tools with which to support individuals with challenging behaviour towards positive behaviour. It is critical that carers do not just hand out reward without seriously reflecting why they are doing it. In order for care workers to maximise the use of reward or positive reinforcers they should do so appropriately:

- Using the praise effort: teachers always say to children, "…Well tried…you did not succeed this time…better luck next time…"

This way the teacher has thought about the effort of the child and encourages them through praise to try again and that they will succeed next time. Similarly in care work the individual should be praised and encouraged to try again towards positive behaviour. A positive reinforcer is thereby seen in "praising the effort".

- Using consistency in rewarding where behaviour has become positive develops a chain or relational link, so that the individual begins to connect the "reward they get with the behaviour". The carer must be consistent and ensure that no confusion is ever derived out of misplaced reward.

- Using specification: In school a child learns through the teachers' specification. The children in my childcare setting do routines, like when they arrive at the setting, they will be welcomed by the teacher. The children over time learn to hand their own courts and place their lunch bags on the rack; they get into class and do free-play and at this they can paint, look at books, play with toys, etc. for ten minutes.

Then the teacher starts a welcome nursery rhyme which is a signal to: "Use it, clean it, and put it away...nicely."

Then the children sit in a circle; it is here that the teacher rewards, by calling each child's name and saying, "Well done, J, you have done good sitting." This goes on until all children in the circle are named and praised. The thanking is repeated exactly, specifically using the same verbal words.

Therefore the importance of positive reinforcement is that it provides the carer with one of the powerful tools with which to support individuals with challenging behaviour towards the effect to have positive behaviour.

Effects of reinforcers on behaviour:

The reinforcers are in themselves tools that enable the individual to be supported, through how they appreciate the reward: the appreciation of the individual for the reward is the effect.

- Reducing challenging behaviour: The target, the certain aim of supported care, is to achieve reduction of challenging behaviour. If a positive reinforcer achieves this target then the carer's job is well done. Therefore, this augments reasons for use of reinforcers.

- Increasing critical ability: with positive reinforcers the individual/client increases in abilities including critical skills such as making choices, waiting their turn, and so on.

- Self-esteem increase: positive reinforcers help individuals make choices, and as they make choices, they increase in critical skills and suddenly the self-esteem begins to rise, and this impacts on the positive achievement of good behaviour.

- Making more effort: improving behaviour takes time, but with the help of positive reinforcers and the support towards positive behaviour the individual will begin to put more effort into recovery ways; these being rewarded becomes a stimulant, something to work towards.

Whilst the importance of positive reinforcement is that it provides the carer with one of the powerful tools with which to support individuals with challenging behaviour towards the effect to have positive behaviour, it is also important for carers to be aware that "positive reinforcers work in two particular contexts, namely; the physical and social factors that affect behaviour":

1. The physical factors that affect behaviour:

This study stipulates that the following physical factors affect behaviour in particular with individuals with challenging behaviour: being hungry, being in pain, having or experiencing thirst, the lacking of sufficient rest or sleep, getting side effects from medication, suffering sensory issues/impairments, interventions from medical staff such as blood tests or administration of injections, and in many instances the need for a toilet. Therefore, whilst the importance of positive reinforcement is that it provides the carer with one of the powerful tools with which to support individuals with challenging behaviour towards the effect to have positive behaviour, it is also important for carers to be aware that positive reinforcers work in physical factors as set out above.

2. The social factors that affect behaviour:

The social factors that affect the behaviour of individuals with challenging behaviour are of a wide range including:

- The loss of control is an effect that affects behaviour: where the individual loses charge of their lives, they escalate in behaviour that challenges.

- Cold or hot temperature: this causes negative effects and the individual feels they either want to be in different clothing.

- Noisy surroundings or environment, including being spoken to too loudly

- Being bored, maybe with inactivity, but also routine, lacking stimulus

- Loneliness, caused by lack of preferred company, or isolation

- Cultural misunderstandings due to values or beliefs

- Overcrowding: individuals with behaviour that challenges can be overwhelmed and agitated by crowds.

- Lights can cause negative effect, where there is very bright or dimmed or flashing lighting that can affect behaviour.

Whilst the importance of positive reinforcement is that it provides the carer with one of the powerful tools with which to support individuals with challenging behaviour towards the effect to have positive behaviour; it is also important for carers to be aware that positive reinforcers work in a social context as set out here.

This has provided a detailed overview of the term "positive reinforcement" and recognising the importance of such in promoting and maintaining positive behaviour.

Avoid confrontation with someone who is emotionally agitated.

In care, there are mechanisms of support systems that carers must use to avoid confrontation with those they care for who become emotionally charged and agitated: to avoid confrontation with someone who is emotionally agitated requires the carer to apply skills learned, such that the carer resists the confrontational behaviour coming from an individual that is highly charged emotionally and seeks a physical confrontation which is usually preceded by verbal and facial violent expressions: confrontation from individuals with challenging behaviour makes them hostile and are attacking carers verbally and physically. The carer has to prepare, predict, and suspect that this kind of behaviour may occur; part of the preparation is the training the carer got. It is important for the carer:

- To know the client/individual that they are going to care for; usually information is on the support plan

- To know what type of behavioural traits the individual has

- To identify the possible triggers that may cause confrontation from the individual which could cause him/her to:

1. Start spitting

2. Start using abusive or threatening words

3. Start screaming and shouting

4. Start directing a pointed finger at carers or anyone present

5. Start self-harming such as pulling own hair, etc.

Once the carer begins to see any of these tendencies, then the carer must ensure that the support plan strategies to help manage the situation are applied. This will help to avoid confrontation. Therefore the carers would take precautions to support the individual by avoiding to:

- Put that individual in the same place as another person for whom they have taken a dislike; for instance, children usually may dislike an individual and wherever they find that individual they begin crying.

- Put things they dislike in their presence

- Offering foods or drinks they dislike. In my family, my child with autism refuses completely anything to do with rice; just the smell of cooking rice is enough to cause tantrums.

- Put them in places where there is no direct care or supervision

- Put them in isolation where they will feel abandoned

- Do things for them, such that decisions are not made by them, so they feel dictated to, powerless, and disrespected

When carers avoid these situations, the triggers towards challenging behaviour which may be confrontational are minimised and managed. Therefore, there are mechanisms of a support system that carers must use to avoid confrontation with those they care for who become emotionally charged and agitated.

To avoid confrontation the carer must use the support systems. The systems promoted by carer scholars are:

a). Techniques of distraction are a good and proven strategy to draw attention of the emotionally agitated individual into something that may calm them down. Among these are things like providing something they would take to or like, show a picture they always like, or talk to them about something good about to happen. In childcare we use this strategy if a child is crying if they are missing their mum; we could start several pleasantries like sing a song, show a toy, and so on. This will normally work well.

b). Avoidance steps: Carers can take steps to help support the individual in avoiding agitation which leads to confrontation. The strategies to follow are primarily to monitor or observe and watch out for the first signs of change in mood or behaviour; this way the carer would then identify any triggers and take supportive action to manage the behaviour, e.g. if the room temperature was high to turn down the heating, or provide a coolant, etc. This way, the confrontation is managed by avoidance of not letting the trigger continue escalating the behaviour.

c). De-escalating strategies: Strategies are applied, but they must be appropriate for the situation. To de-escalate strategies will help the avoidance of confrontation and this study gives the example of simply, talk to the individual and tell them firmly but nicely to "stop" when they are showing the first sign of agitation, or ask them what the matter is, and if they have verbal communication they will tell you. This way, the confrontation is managed and de-escalated.

d). The carer can use assertive methods of communication, so that the individual whilst being confrontational can still understand that that behaviour will not be tolerated, it is unwanted, and they should stop it. Whilst doing this it must be said calmly without shouting or aggression. This is effective with a display of willingness to help; the carer asking the individual what it is that is bothering them. This way, the confrontation is managed.

e). Allowing space and time: Carers working to avoid confrontation must allow space, and that space could be ensuring that the right environment is there. Maybe the individual would prefer for a period to go outside the building for a walk. The time is ensuring the routines are maintained and consistent. One suggestion by this course is to practice "breathing exercises". This way, the confrontation can be avoided and is managed for people with challenging behaviour.

f). Getting other people involved: Carers would do well not to be alone especially when the individual is confrontational. This helps the safety of the client as well as for the carer. It is also useful if the carer's family member can come around, to help pacify the agitation. This way, the confrontation is managed.

g). Staying calm as a carer: this is critical to success and is the tool that enables the carer to do the job.

When calm one can recollect all strategies necessary and can refer to the support plan. When calm the carer can speak to the individual calmly. When calm the carer can call colleagues for assistance and take all necessary steps. Above all when the individual with challenging behaviour tries confrontation and gets back a calm response, they are psychologically deflated, but also see that there is an offer to get what they want. This way, the confrontation is managed.

h). Identifying the causes of confrontation will help the carer to respond appropriately. For instance if the individual is affected by loud noise coming through an open window, once identified, the closure of the window will de-escalate the behaviour. Some instances may be a radio or television. This way, the confrontation is managed.

Therefore, in care practice, there are mechanisms of a support system that carers must use to avoid confrontation with those they care for who become emotionally charged and agitated.

The challenge to describe how using knowledge of the individual can help to manage behaviour:

Using knowledge of the individual can help to manage behaviour that challenges: person-centred support results from person-centred planning of care. This is why the support plan is central to the carers' knowledge: that plan contains the personal details, the issues, the triggers, the professionals that care for the individual, and the family or advocate's contacts.

Knowing the individual means focussing the care on the person, making the service person-centric, in ensuring managing challenging behaviour using the support plan. This will ensure that the personality and the risks around the client are well assessed, so the individual is cared for with dignity and accorded appropriate respect.

1. The carer's knowledge of the individual helps ensure that the individual feels valued and listened to.

2. The carer's knowledge of the individual helps ensure that where communication disorders exist, the individual has a method of communicating effectively.

3. The carer's knowledge of the individual helps to give the individual other ways of communicating a need.

4. The carer's knowledge of the individual helps reduce, where necessary, expectations of the individual and of care staff.

5. The carer's knowledge of the individual helps determine triggers in the environment, such as noise or attitudes and beliefs in carers that might provoke or maintain challenging behaviour.

6. The carer's knowledge of the individual helps the individual him/herself and their carers to recognise distress.

7. The carer's knowledge of the individual helps develop the individual's coping strategies for dealing with problems.

8. The carer's knowledge of the individual helps anticipate potential problems and intervene where appropriate (for example, by providing additional support, redirection to another activity, or reducing noise level).

9. The carer's knowledge of the individual helps training and support for care staff in prevention and management of problems.

10. Care staff sharing knowledge and expertise.

These strategies must be used to ensure that the individual is not agitated, distressed, or humiliated. Therefore, through the above points the care will be person-centred care: if the carers fail to use person-centred care, the individual's quality of life could deteriorate and the escalation in behaviour that challenges will reach difficult proportions. Therefore, the person-centred care is all-important as the route to knowing the client and giving them appropriate support. Person-centred support results from person-centred planning of care for the individual. The family, friends, and professionals are to be engaged and agreed in the planning when it is being drawn up.

The challenge to agree on the strategies for management of behaviour:

From agreed strategies carers begin knowing the individual; which means focussing the care on the client, making the service person-centric using those agreed strategies, by ensuring managing challenging behaviour using the support plan. This will ensure that the personality and the risks around the client are well assessed, so the individual is cared for with dignity and accorded appropriate respect. To have agreed strategies of management of behaviour that challenges meets the following areas:

It provides the information required to know the individual/client.

It must be a collective and multi-agency approach.

It is the most important part of planning care.

It outlines and sustains the consistency required in care.

It helps with the routines of the individual.

It helps that all who work with the individual know the individual and know what to expect, or can predict triggers but also know how to work with the individual.

"Give her, her dummy…when she shows she wants to sleep otherwise she will not," says Mum to the carer in the pre-school childcare; so that the same routine, soother, is used both at home and in the childcare setting. This maintains routine as would be at home. Therefore the planning must be done by all involved in the care of an individual. This is the multi-agency approach.

Multi-Agency Working:

The multi-agency approach is the pooling or gathering together of representatives of all the agencies or professions and family to work or to discuss the care plan, to work out strategies of care to help the "knowing of the individual", to help manage their behaviour; these agencies could include:

- Family and/or friends

- Advocates in cases where there are no immediate relatives/family

- Social services

- Schools or other education and learning agencies and departments

- Young people's welfare and clubs/groups

- Healthcare centres/agents which will include: psychologists, psychiatrists, physiotherapists, occupational therapists, speech and language therapists, audiologists, and any other health workers that are relevant to the condition of the individual.

- Day centres, including respite or residential homes

Multi-agency working brings in advantages:

Multi agency approaches in care bring about advantages of knowing the individual and in every area of care means focussing the care on the person, making the service person-centric, in ensuring managing challenging behaviour using the support plan. This will ensure that the personality and the risks around the client are well assessed, so the individual is cared for with dignity and accorded appropriate respect.

The advantages of multi-agency are:

1. Coordination of care: The agencies use either meetings or electronic communication to share information, so at a glance the professionals and family, at a click of a button, can see what updates are made regarding the behaviour of an individual. This makes coordinated care smooth between carers.

2. Holistic care delivery: for clients that may have complicated needs, this enables the various professionals to coordinate and care for the individual, and as the carers link up in a holistic way, this minimises the likelihood of triggers and can enable individuals towards positive behaviour.

3. Any new complications are prevented: The multi-agency approach to care will usually minimise problems such as medicine side effects causing triggers without the warning to the carer. Any new issues are shared by the professionals and action is taken ensuring avoidance of problems that lead to escalated behaviour.

The multi-agency approach helps build capacity to know the individual for all who work with the client: knowing the individual means focussing the care on the person, making the service person-centric, in ensuring managing challenging behaviour using the support plan. This will ensure that the personality and the risks around the client are well assessed, so the individual is cared for with dignity and accorded appropriate respect. However there are also some disadvantages in multi-agency working such as the following:

Multi-agency work disadvantages in care:

1. It is time-consuming: There are always issues that arise with management of time as different carers will have personal issues which they juggle with their job of care. Understanding and cooperation is essential to allow for delegates/representatives to be in meetings on behalf of.

2. Budgets may cause friction: Some departments or sections of care have limited budgets and this can cause difficulties for some to be part of the multi-agency. Where this disadvantage occurs understanding is critical; for instance many advocacy agencies are voluntary or charitable and may depend on volunteers.

However, overall we learn that multi-agency work helps us. Knowing the individual means focussing the care on the person, making the service person-centric, in ensuring managing challenging behaviour using the support plan. This will ensure that the personality and the risks around the client are well assessed, so the individual is cared for with dignity and accorded appropriate respect.

3. The management of time: There is always the need to have some form of communication or meeting, either by telephone conferencing, Skype, or direct face to face in order to discuss and agree any strategies for the individual. Time is a factor, and getting all individuals at the same time in one place may be difficult, in view of the demands on services. Whilst disadvantageous, it is not insurmountable to coordinate and manage time given the various ways meetings can be held and information exchanged.

The above has provided a good explanation of how being knowledgeable surrounding an individual's behaviours as a care worker is beneficial in providing support tailored to their needs. This is essential as by not doing so, this could contribute to an increase in challenging behaviour.

CHAPTER 11

The challenge of how to maintain the dignity of individuals when responding to incidents of challenging behaviour:

RESPECT AND DIGNITY ARE CRITICAL:

Maintain the client, child, or individual's dignity:

For carers to maintain the dignity of an individual when responding to incidents of behaviour that challenges, the carers need to understand that "dignity is respect and value mingled together": the carer will maintain the individual's dignity by making the individual feel valuable, worthy, and respected. To maintain dignity is to treat the client uniquely as a person; the issues or needs they have are personal and therefore must be treated with a person-centred care plan and strategies that are responsible and respectful.

- Therefore, to maintain dignity of the individual, carers should be providing privacy, e.g. create a bit of seclusion and remove other individuals when discussing the health issues of the individual.

- To promote dignity or preserve it the carer should speak with respect and calmly to the individual.

- The carer to maintain dignity must not shout.

- To maintain the dignity of the individual the carer must ask them to cooperate in the care, basically requesting.

- The carer should not tell the individual what to do; rather it is best to inform them about what the carer is doing, how, and why.

This book as a study enables us to avoid the pitfalls of treating individuals in a derisory manner; therefore a carer must not deal with an individual in:

An angry way; be abusive or abrupt; the individual needs care and attention not bullying.

A humiliating manner, not valuing the person or the individual in any way; the individual has issues that need care, not humiliation.

A way that lowers the self-esteem, self-worth, or confidence of the client who has challenging behaviour.

A manner that could increase or intensify challenging behaviour; this individual needs support towards positive behaviour.

In a way that distresses the individual.

In a way that can cause or increase feelings of isolation.

In a way that can make the individual self-harm.

In a way that will make the individual turn to drugs or abuse medication.

Therefore, to maintain dignity is to treat the client uniquely as a person. The issues or needs they have are personal and therefore must be treated with a person-centred care plan and strategies that are responsible and respectful.

The carer must use the following strategies:

- Uphold a lower-levelled tone of voice: The carer must ensure they are speaking in a low tone, not patronising, but respectful and not shouting. Due respect must continue to maintain the dignity of the individual. This will contribute greatly towards defusing challenging behaviour. This is how to maintain the dignity of individuals when responding to incidents of behaviour that challenges.

- Maintaining a non-aggressive posture: The carer's way of standing, the eye contact, the expressions and gestures must show the individual that the carer is there to support, to help, and is not being aggressive. The carer must avoid shouting or pointing in the face of the individual. This will contribute greatly towards defusing challenging behaviour. This is how to maintain the dignity of individuals when responding to incidents of behaviour that challenges.

- Respectfully addressing the client/individual: Culture here plays some part. Words like "you" could sound demeaning, so appropriate words should be used, e.g. the name of the individual. This will contribute greatly towards defusing challenging behaviour. This is how to maintain the dignity of individuals when responding to incidents of behaviour that challenges.

- Empathy and support should be offered: The carer in supporting the individual can also show understanding and empathy, but not becoming emotional. The individual will feel secure when they know the carer comprehends what's going on, what's causing the behaviour. This will contribute greatly towards defusing challenging behaviour. This is how to maintain the dignity of individuals when responding to incidents of behaviour that challenges.

- Maintain complete non-judgement: If carers have pre-conceived and biased judgement of issues before contact with the individual, there would be a blanking out of the person-centred approach, therefore it is better not to have judgements which would result in the disrespect of the individual. The individual's views matter. This will contribute greatly towards defusing challenging behaviour. This is how to maintain the dignity of individuals when responding to incidents of behaviour that challenges.

- Making the individual decent: In many cases of escalated behaviour, individuals may tear clothing. The carer's role is to support the individual towards positive behaviour; it is important to help ensure the modesty of the individual where appropriate. And the carer must ensure their own safety if the situation is volatile. However, covering the individual discreetly and properly ensures their dignity. This will contribute greatly towards defusing challenging behaviour. This is how to maintain the dignity of individuals when responding to incidents of behaviour that challenges.

- Make the individual feel valued: Carers must uplift the morale of the individual as part of the support. The work is not to merely observe, but to enable the increase of self-esteem and self-worth in the individual. This will contribute greatly towards defusing challenging behaviour. This is how to maintain the dignity of individuals when responding to incidents of behaviour that challenges.

- The cause of the behaviour: The carers have to deal with the trigger, ensuring they identify and address the cause of the behaviour. Usually the source of the behaviour if dealt with may help secure immediate recovery towards positive behaviour. This will contribute greatly towards defusing challenging behaviour. This is how to maintain the dignity of individuals when responding to incidents of behaviour that challenges.

- Supporting the client/individual with control: The carer must help in all aspects to enable the individual to retain the feeling of being in control of their own life, show that the individual is a responsible individual; this is part of ensuring dignity and respecting the client. It leads to the individual becoming more confident, regaining self-worth and self-esteem. This will contribute greatly towards defusing challenging behaviour. This is how to maintain the dignity of individuals when responding to incidents of behaviour that challenges.

- Carers being, remaining, calm and collected: The carer controls him/herself, so they have no visible emotional involvement with the challenging behaviour they are faced with. To ensure good observation and support, plus setting an example, requires the carer to remain calm, deal with the individual appropriately, and call in support as necessary. This is how to maintain the dignity of individuals when responding to incidents of behaviour that challenges.

By not ensuring dignity an individual may display negative behaviours such as anger, distress, feelings of isolation, and there may be increased signs of mental illness as you correctly point out.

Examples of different techniques that are used to defuse behaviour that challenges:

There are examples of different techniques that are used to defuse behaviour that challenges; where there is a need to defuse a situation, the carer will have a number of options of techniques. These examples are known as effective and positive support systems: there are successful and unsuccessful techniques, and when one fails there is always an alternative to defuse the situation. These systems support the emotions and maintenance of the quality of life whilst preserving the dignity of the individual with behaviour that challenges. This system involves some of the strategies set out hereunder; however, prior to using the techniques it has to be stated that the carer must be equipped with the right skills to harness the following strategies:

Techniques to defuse escalating behaviour:

- Carers being, remaining, calm and collected is part and parcel of the job: The carer controls him/herself, so that they have no visible emotional involvement with the challenging behaviour they are faced with. To ensure good observation and support, plus setting an example, requires the carer to remain calm, deal with the individual appropriately, and call in support as necessary.

- Techniques of diversion: If applied early, diversion can support the individual and defuse the behaviour. When the carer works to intervene using diversionary techniques this distracts the individuals from the escalation and they fix their attention on the diversion; this can help defuse behaviour that challenges.

- Techniques of crisis management: Action, action, action; immediate and or prompt action has to be employed, so that the situation is arrested. Usually the care support plan will provide a step-by-step strategy to be put into place, when the situation or the escalation of behaviour is at break-point. This has to be managed without panic or anxiety from the part of the carer.

- Measures of prevention: Preventing behaviour from happening or escalating is highlighted as the best technique in defusing challenging behaviour. The carer needs to observe and monitor, ensuring suitability of the environment and surroundings of where the individual is, but also be equipped and use appropriate strategies to prevent triggers from happening. This will defuse behaviour that challenges.

- Seeking support: Self-safety for carers is very important, but also competency is not just about dealing with the individual and doing what one can, it is about predicting or gauging that the situation is such; I, the carer, need support, to call on colleagues or other professionals who are more competent to respond to the behaviour that challenges. This technique can defuse the situation as appropriate support will be drawn in.

- Application of the person-centred techniques: The dignity of the individual with challenging behaviour is central to management and supporting behaviour, therefore the support plan in place must be referred to sustain the way the individual is dealt with. This will ensure their particular way of communication and all the other relevant things that centre on the individual's person. When dealt with as a person, an individual with due respect, this will contribute to defusing the behaviour that challenges.

- To realise by acknowledgement the carer's own limitation and competence: Abilities depend on a number of factors including specific skills, therefore a carer who acknowledges their own competencies and limitations will work in a consultative manner and multi-agency network with a pool of other carers to call upon in case the situation is beyond this carer's abilities and capacity to handle. This helps in defusing the behaviour from escalation as the competent, able professional will come to support the individual.

The unsuccessful techniques:

There are unsuccessful techniques when attempting to defuse behaviour that challenges. Every individual is different, that is why a person-centred plan and approach is essential. When strategies or techniques fail to control the triggers, the carer can employ alternatives, for instance: the individual's behaviour begins to escalate; the carer refers to the care plan where the first suggested strategy to control triggers is "diversionary technique". If it fails, the behaviour continues to escalate...the carer stops the diversion after a number of recommended attempts. The care plan suggests "changing the environment". The carer looks at the room temperature, and it's above the twenty-degree mark, so the carer reduces the temperature to the eighteen-degree mark and waits five minutes. The individual is now managing slowly to calm down!

There are several strategies that fail to work, but the carer has to keep alternating until the correct technique is found.

When found, the correct technique helps in defusing the behaviour from escalation as the competent, able professional will come to support the individual.

Significance of avoiding self-risk:

As carers provide support for behaviour, it is not unusual for physical injury to occur to them:

- The carer is at the frontline of behaviour that challenges. When individuals want to be aggressive, they could target not only equipment around them, but also attack carers verbally and in instances physically, either throwing objects or aiming hands to punch. Carers have to have the training of dealing with such physical injury or harm when it happens to themselves or the individual through self-harm. Many times the individual may unintentionally cause injury to the carer.

- The carer must also be aware of emotional effects, where the carer is at risk of emotional burnout; this would be the result of regularly encountering distressing behaviour. The carer must have safeguards, like time off work and break time at work, debriefing sessions. The carer will have training of when to seek support if emotional issues are rising.

Knowing these issues is important and this will contribute to defusing the behaviour that challenges, and competent staff will be called in to defuse the behaviour from escalation as those competent, able professionals will come to support the individual.

Physical Interventions:

The defusing of behaviour that challenges is a challenge to the carer. To defuse the behaviour may require physical interventions:

The carer must know that physical interventions are intended only where the need is that the situation must be put under prompt control. The immediate control arises only if there is likelihood of self-harm or injury to others, including the carer. Physical intervention may take the nature of restricting the body movement of the individual, using restraints which are recommended under specific conditions and specific guidelines. There are prescribed interventions to use restraints policies in care settings. This study suggests that the physical restraints should only be:

- Necessary to the behaviour

- Reasonable to the behaviour

- Proportionate to the behaviour

- Used or administered/conducted by staff trained on using restraints

- Additional to other strategies of de-escalating the behaviour

- Least restrictive to the individual as necessary and for a short time

- Used to control the individual whilst s/he is being monitored and observed

And a record of the matter should be done immediately and detail why it was necessary. Physical interventions may therefore help in defusing the behaviour from escalation as an addition or combination to other strategies and the competent, able professional must support the individual, ensuring ethical and legal compliance.

The above information has demonstrated a good understanding of a range of techniques that could be used to defuse challenging behaviour and you touch upon crisis prevention. Below is provided an interesting web link that discusses behaviour management strategies and crisis intervention.

https://www.crisisprevention.com/Blog/August-2012/Behavior-Management-Strategies

The challenge to review how a carer's own actions can defuse or exacerbate an individual's behaviour:

The carer must be aware of how his/her own actions maintain the dignity of the individual: it depends on the nature of actions that the carers take. The carer must consider:

- Am I self-aware? I.e. am I the right carer to provide this care for this individual?

- Have I the equipment necessary?

- Have I got support such as supervision or colleagues that I can call on?

- Are the actions I am taking appropriate?

- Am I sitting or standing in the right place?

- Am I using the right posture, language, gestures?

Every individual is different, and the carer should be self-aware about how to respond or deal with that individual in a person-centred approach, using appropriate actions: through self-awareness the carer can use the following to defuse behaviour or prevent it from starting:

- The approach must be person-centred

- Maintain the dignity of the individual

- Avoiding any triggers from the outset of approaching the individual

- Refer to the care support plan for the individual to use the outlined strategies to help the individual's behaviour

- Use distraction techniques

- Communicating positively and assertively with the individual

- Ensuring to remain calm, as much as the individual may be behaving challengingly

To be self-aware the carer must therefore ensure to avoid the actions and things that could exacerbate challenging behaviour in an individual, including the following:

- If the carer panics the behaviour of the individual would be exacerbated

- The carer shouting

- The carer using inappropriate posture and gestures such as pointing

- If the carer uses techniques they are not trained to use

- Where the carer fails to use the individual's care support plan

- If the carer used inappropriate intervention including restraint techniques

- Failure to uphold the individual's dignity

- Not using the preferred communication language of the individual

- If the carer humiliates the individual

These points of self-awareness should be an element that helps the carer, to avoid escalating or exacerbating the challenging behaviour of an individual. This then shows how significant the carer's own "self-awareness" is in controlling the situation.

The significance of the carer's self-awareness:

As a practitioner it is good practice if a carer:

- Examines and deals with any "professional, practice, or career developmental needs". This in my industry of childcare is constant as there are always new and better ways of caring for children, and regular training helps us in updating staff knowledge.

- Examines any unmet or unfulfilled competence training.

- Examines own carer practices through reflecting on practice and overall conduct when caring. When the carer reflects and deals with their own professional competence they are better able to identify and deal with any self would-be triggers to behavioural challenges.

Therefore the significance of a carer's self-awareness can defuse behaviour from escalating. Self-reflection is important:

In the childcare industry we reflect through day-to-day self-evaluation as we care for children. This reflection or self-evaluation is done as follows:

- Carers will write down on forms known as "trackers" for each child any observations, how the child is responding to care, learning, or play. This writing or recording is done instantly or immediately when things occur.

- Carers keep learning journals for the individual child; we also ensure there is a register for attendance, and we regularly record observations and review those records.

- In childcare we get local authority staff to observe what happens in specific situations, and then this is fed back to all carers. We also go through annual/biannual Ofsted inspections giving objective opinions and being critical of the standard of care delivery.

- Carers can ask for informal supervision; this helps where there are new amendments to monitor, and examines their effectiveness.

Therefore self-reflection is important to maintain and improve the standards of care delivered by the carer. There are benefits that accrue if the reflector, i.e. carer, is reflecting genuinely from the betterment of care and how they deliver it: the following benefits can accrue:

New strategies:

When recorded, written down, they are learned quickly and tested and remembered. Best practice: this is when those new strategies are part of any improvement that can accrue from self-reflection.

Evidencing work: Reflective practice helps carers in all situations, so that where reporting is due, it can be done effectively using accurate information that was recorded when the event occurred. Therefore self-awareness and the added in component of self-reflection can defuse behaviour from escalating.

This section of the chapter has so far provided a good use of examples to show how situations can be diffused or exacerbated. It is extremely important as a professional carer to recognise the impact your approach, tone, body language, and communication have on an individual. Workers should have a good level of self-awareness to ensure they are able to appropriately respond to individuals at all times. Failure to do so would seek to exacerbate challenging behaviour.

CHAPTER 12

The role of others in supporting individuals who exhibit behaviour that is perceived as challenging

THE CHALLENGE IS KNOWING THE REFERRAL SERVICES AVAILABLE TO PROVIDE SUPPORT FOR CHILDREN OR ADULT INDIVIDUALS

The referral services available to provide support for individuals:

A referral service is usually a place for better care where an individual would be sent to; in other words where they are signposted to: this signposting or referral occurs where the immediate or first point, e.g. a local doctor, is unable to deal with the situation, or the individual's needs require advanced care.

Therefore, the individual can start the chain of referral services by:

- The individual him/herself goes to the doctor because they are unable to deal with the situation themselves.

- The family can take the individual to a doctor when the family cannot meet the needs of the individual.

- The doctor can refer the individual to a hospital or specialised unit.

- Social services welfare departments can refer the individual to hospital where there are signs of potential self-harm or risk of violence to others.

In childcare we work closely with social services especially when caring for children with particular special needs. Social services and Ofsted help in the monitoring of learning and safeguarding of vulnerable children.

The arrangement for a referral: depending on what the needs are the referral can be arranged by any of the following:

- A general practitioner; a doctor who normally treats the individual when unwell can refer to a better equipped facility

- A teacher when there is a situation, e.g. in school (Parents have to work closely with teachers where children have special learning plans and behaviour issues.)

- Health visitors (Home visiting nurses help make referrals all the time to AE or speech and language for children.)

- Health professionals

- The police in their work find individuals, e.g. on the street, in a shopping centre, who have suffered mental breakdown and have to make appropriate referrals to social services or hospitals

Therefore, there is a range of services where individuals who pose challenging behaviour can be referred.

These services will range from the following:

Who will individuals be referred to?

1) Education psychologist: The child that has special needs may need an education psychologist, and this is made by the teachers where the child attends. The child in adolescence, aged from ten to nineteen, can benefit from support on education, emotional, and social issues, through talking and listening, identifying the strategies to manage any needs and learning issues the child finds which cause that child emotional and social difficulties.

2) Clinical psychologist to deal with difficulties of social and emotional nature. There may be issues of learning, issues of substance abuse, and social complications that the individual cannot cope with, where the clinical psychologist will help.

3) Nutritionist: who specialises in food and nutrition. Many times children and adults who have difficulties dealing with food and suffer eating disorders need advice and guidance on how to cope with food.

4) Psychiatrist: Where mental illness is the issue, usually the referral will be made to a psychiatrist who will observe, examine, and deal with the issues that trigger the behaviour that challenges. Identifying triggers and causes of difficulties can be identified by a behaviour therapist in the psychiatry discipline.

5) Speech and language therapists: Communication being crucial to social interaction, if

individuals have poor on no communication they would be referred to speech and language therapists to help in the development of language. Small children who reach the age of speech but lack it are usually referred to this service. In my childcare setting we frequently have to accommodate the visits of individual children from "speech and language" therapists who are helping the development of a child.

6) Behaviour therapist: to change harmful or self-destructive behaviour of an individual a behaviour therapist will help with identifying issues, social, emotional, or mental, that cause challenging behaviour and provide calming and appropriate treatment recommendations.

7) Physiotherapist: musculoskeletal injuries suffered by individuals need to be helped to repair, and the physiotherapist can help with mobility and flexibility of muscle and bones to repair any damage that may have occurred with the individual

8) Occupational therapist: daily activities make individuals independent; the failure to be able to do simple tasks can occur as a result of underlying issues, which occupational therapy helps rectify.

9) Social services: for the safeguarding and welfare of community/public social services; they are also especially concerned with issues affecting children. Social services ensure all other agencies or departments that have a duty to care are providing it. Individuals or others can refer to social services to have needs addressed.

10). Counselling: Where the individual may need some guidance, being listened to, when spoilt for choice or having none at all, the counselling service helps as they will be non-judgemental. Counsellors assist if behavioural triggers are not identified; they become apparent when someone listens neutrally to the individual.

Therefore, it is important for a carer to be aware of all the referral services available to provide support for individuals.

The above is fantastic information that any parent, carer, or teacher will be able to harness: the book so far correctly defined what is meant by a referral agency and provided a range of examples of professionals who may be involved with an individual who displays behaviour that challenges. The chapter so far has provided clear explanation of each role demonstrating an excellent understanding of the support that can be offered.

LIMITATIONS AND ACCOUNTABILITIES WHEN SUPPORTING INDIVIDUALS EXHIBITING CHALLENGING BEHAVIOUR:

There are limitations and accountabilities when supporting individuals exhibiting behaviour that is perceived as challenging. What this means is that a carer can deal with certain aspects of behaviour, but also a carer is unable to deal with certain others. Using the self-awareness technique the carer is able to self-reflect and ascertain what they are capable of and what is beyond their capability, not just so, but also knowing that a dentist is not a surgeon and in my childcare setting this is such that Mum is not Dad. Through self-awareness and self-reflection carers become more focussed and robust in mannerism and methodology, using strategies appropriately.

The limitations and accountabilities for a carer:

It is a limitation where the carer is unskilled to do a certain care element, whereas it is an accountability as the carer carries out interventions; they could be trained or not, have the skill or not; they are accountable. On reflection, should they have intervened? With hindsight, have they overstepped the mark?

- Therefore carers working in a network of professionals always know when and where to call on other colleagues to help support interventions in situations of challenging behaviour.

- Carers know how and who to make referrals to for an individual with challenging behaviour, as the carer is accountable for any failings or success for the behaviour of the individual in a situation.

- Whilst risk-taking is possible, but consultation with supervisors helps to avert unnecessary trauma which could result out of risk-taking, as a carer, know your limits.

Therefore, in the childcare industry, "Family expect everyone responsible for their relative who is a child, son, or daughter's carer to be able to make the right decisions that are genuinely in the best interests of the child."

To counter limitations whilst upholding accountabilities in childcare, we uphold that the importance of effective training is as follows:

Effective Training for Child-Carers Helps to Prevent Failure:

In care and teaching, the effective teacher training helps prepare new teachers for the challenges in childcare or teaching.

- It can help teachers and carers feel more confident about many common problems that arise for teachers each day.

- Without this background of effective training carers and or teachers might feel like failures and eventually give up.

Effective Training Helps Avoid Teacher Burnout:

- Effective carer and teacher training programs will address self-awareness and help carer or teacher burnout.

- In the first instance, it helps new carers and teachers to understand what can lead to carer or teacher burnout.

- In the second instance or some cases, burning out is just the stress of daily teaching.

- Thirdly, burning out can also be caused by not varying the information and methods of caring or teaching enough.

- Carer training programs that focus on particular subject areas like social studies or mathematics can help students learn about different ways in which a subject can be presented.

Effective Carer Training Provides an Understanding of the Benchmarks for Achievement:

- Carers who are inexperienced in behaviour support focus on getting individuals to calm down in cases of challenging behaviour, but fail to enable the individual to continually self-support.

- In childcare we have to ensure the carer or teacher is not just supporting children to memorize and regurgitate success because it does not show true individual child achievement?

- Without a background to what does and does not constitute authentic care or child learning, new carers or teachers sometimes create situations or lessons that don't lead to the results they were expecting.

- However, childcare preparation programs can help students understand how to find and apply effective benchmarks for student achievement.

Effective Training Provides Supported Practice in a Controlled Environment:

- When it comes to childcare, reading a book or playing with a toy is not enough. Even hearing child-carers talk about childcare and teaching methods is not enough.

- A carer in any area needs practice to relate to children, teaching combined with effective mentoring in order to help them understand what is required from them in their carer position.

- It is imperative that carers, when learning to care, are placed in appropriate care situations that meet their interests.

- Further, the supervising trainer must be involved and provide feedback each day to help student carers learn.

Effective Training Helps to Stop Costly Experimenting on Individuals or Children in Childcare

- Carers must never experiment with new techniques that they have not been trained on.

- Carers without proper training could easily try things that a trainer might have taught them would not work.

- This experimenting comes at a cost in terms of care learning, as most experienced carers would know.

- It is very easy to fail individuals who suffer challenging behaviour if a carer exhibits incompetence, unfairness, and inconsistency from the beginning.

- The carer without appropriate training risks losing respect and interest. The ultimate cost of this failure is in what the individual or client will not achieve; i.e. full potential.

Effective training is important:

Like childcare, health and social care require effective training so that appropriate strategies are learned and applied by the carer who has been trained. The training offers the carer the range and variety of options and a trained carer will be governed by the person-centred care support plan. This study gives an example where the individual with behaviour that challenges can be sedated instead of being put into restraints. The client has a choice and if the carer does not take into account the client's preference, there could be trauma and anxiety resulting in exacerbated behaviour. The carer's training will therefore enhance the carer's competence and skills as they will learn:

- About making good judgements, making risk assessment of the situation prior to intervention

- The tactics of self-defence if they are physically attacked by an individual with challenging behaviour

- Knowledge of freeing oneself should they be held or grabbed unexpectedly

- Being aware of the law, the legal accountability when using physical interventions

- Knowing how to use the restraints and when

- Legal and moral aspects of uses of physical interventions

- Being able to make assessment of medical considerations when applying physical interventions

Therefore it is important that care workers should be aware of limitations and accountabilities. Effective training will help the carer understand that there are a number of factors to take into account before taking such action as applying physical interventions:

1. The law: The Human Rights Act 1998 has to be considered to uphold the rights and dignity of the individual if physical intervention or restraints are to be used. Carers should use the least restrictive choice of intervention. The Mental Capacity Act 2005 and/or Mental Capacity Act 2007 can be applied where appropriate to ensure that the individual does not cause self-harm or cause harm to others.

2. Ethical issues: carers through their training should be able to discern if and whether the restraint to be used is correct, right, and justified for the individual with behaviour that challenges.

3. Cultural consideration: Beliefs, values, and culture are personal issues for the individual. Therefore the carers need not be judgemental or assume things. Carers using the care plan will familiarise themselves with the individual and take actions that are appropriate.

4. The environment: The environment is a vast element in the life of an individual and the carer; it is everything that is happening, but also that which is not happening. Carers should be mindful of:

- The area or space they have to work in

- Is the room appropriately lit?

- Are there unnecessary noises from an open window?

- Is there enough room?

The environment is critical, especially when applying physical intervention, especially in cases where individuals may not be willing to have such an intervention applied.

There are limitations and accountabilities when supporting individuals exhibiting behaviour that is perceived as challenging. What this means is that a carer can deal with certain aspects of behaviour, but also a carer is unable to deal with certain others. Using the self-awareness technique the carer is able to self-reflect and ascertain what they are capable of and what is beyond their capability, not just so, but also knowing that a dentist is not a surgeon and in my childcare setting this is such that Mum is not Dad. Through self-awareness and self-reflection carers become more focussed and robust in mannerism and methodology, using strategies appropriately.

The limitations and accountabilities for a carer:

It is a limitation where the carer is unskilled to do a certain care element, whereas it is an accountability as the carer carries out interventions; they could be trained or not, have the skill or not; they are accountable. On reflection, should they have intervened? With hindsight, have they overstepped the mark?

- Therefore a carer working in a network of professionals always knows when and where to call on other colleagues to help support interventions in situations of challenging behaviour.

.

- Carers know how and who to make referrals to for an individual with challenging behaviour, as the carer is accountable for any failings or success for the behaviour of the individual in a situation.

- Whilst risk-taking is possible, but consultation with supervisors helps to avert unnecessary trauma which could result out of risk-taking, as a carer, know your limits. Therefore, in the childcare industry, "Family expect everyone responsible for their relative who is a child, son, or daughter's carer to be able to make the right decisions that are genuinely in the best interests of the child."

To counter limitations whilst upholding accountabilities in childcare, we uphold that the importance of effective training is as follows:

Effective training for child-carers helps to prevent failure:

In care and teaching, the effective teacher training helps prepare new teachers for the challenges in childcare or teaching.

- It can help teachers and carers feel more confident about many common problems that arise for teachers each day.

- Without this background, of effective training, carers and/or teachers might feel like failures and eventually give up.

Effective training helps avoid teacher burnout:

- Effective carer and teacher training programs will address self-awareness and help carer or teacher burnout.

- In the first instance, it helps new carers and teachers to understand what can lead to carer or teacher burnout.

- In the second instance or some cases, burning out is just the stress of daily teaching.

- Thirdly, burning out can also be caused by not varying the information and methods of caring or teaching enough.

- Carer training programs that focus on particular subject areas like social studies or mathematics can help students learn about different ways in which a subject can be presented.

Effective Carer Training Provides an Understanding of the Benchmarks for Achievement.

- Carers who are inexperienced in behaviour support focus on getting individuals to calm down in cases of challenging behaviour, but fail to enable the individual to continually self-support.

- In childcare we have to ensure the carer or teacher is not just supporting children to memorize and regurgitate success because it does not show true individual child achievement?

- Without a background to what does and does not constitute authentic care or child learning, new carers or teachers sometimes create situations or lessons that don't lead to the results they were expecting.

- However, childcare preparation programs can help students understand how to find and apply effective benchmarks for student achievement.

Effective Training Provides Supported Practice in a Controlled Environment

- When it comes to childcare, reading a book or playing with a toy is not enough. Even hearing child-carers talk about childcare and teaching methods is not enough.

- A carer in any area needs practice to relate to children, teaching combined with effective mentoring, in order to help them understand what is required from them in their carer position.

- It is imperative that carers, when learning to care, are placed in appropriate care situations that meet their interests.

- Further, the supervising trainer must be involved and provide feedback each day to help student carers learn.

Effective Training Helps to Stop Costly Experimenting on Individuals or Children in Childcare

- Carers must never experiment with new techniques that they have not been trained on.

- Carers without proper training could easily try things that a trainer might have taught them would not work.

- This experimenting comes at a cost in terms of care learning and most practicing carers would know this.

- It is very easy to fail individuals who suffer challenging behaviour if a carer exhibits incompetence, unfairness, and inconsistency from the beginning.

- The carer without appropriate training risks losing respect and interest. The ultimate cost of this failure is in what the individual or client will not achieve; i.e. full potential.

Effective training is important:

Like childcare, health and social care require effective training so that appropriate strategies are learned and applied by the carer who has been trained. The training offers the carer the range and variety of options and a trained carer will be governed by the person-centred care support plan. This study gives an example where the individual with behaviour that challenges can be sedated instead of being put into restraints. The client has a choice and if the carer does not take into account the client's preference, there could be trauma and anxiety resulting in exacerbated behaviour. Carers' training will therefore enhance the carer's competence and skills as they will learn:

- About making good judgements, making risk assessment of the situation prior to intervention

- The tactics of self-defence if they are physically attacked by an individual with challenging behaviour

- Knowledge of freeing oneself should they be held or grabbed unexpectedly

- Being aware of the law, the legal accountability when using physical interventions

- Knowing how to use the restraints and when

- Legal and moral aspects of uses of physical interventions

- Being able to make assessments of medical considerations when applying physical interventions

Therefore it is important that care workers should be aware of limitations and accountabilities. Effective training will help the carer understand that there are a number of factors to take into account before taking such action as applying physical interventions:

1. The law:

The Human Rights Act 1998 has to be considered to uphold the rights and dignity of the individual if physical intervention or restraints are to be used. Carers should use the least restrictive choice of intervention. The Mental Capacity Act 2005 and/or Mental Capacity Act 2007 can be applied where appropriate to ensure that the individual does not cause self-harm or cause harm to others.

2. Ethical issues:

Carers through their training should be able to discern if and whether the restraint to be used is correct, right, and justified for the individual with behaviour that challenges.

3. Cultural consideration:

Beliefs, values, and culture are personal issues for the individual. Therefore the carers need not be judgemental or assume things. Carers using the care plan will familiarise themselves with the individual and take actions that are appropriate.

4. The environment:

The environment is a vast element in the life of an individual and the carer; it is everything that is happening, but also that which is not happening. Carers should be mindful of:

- The area or space they have to work in

- Is the room appropriately lit?

- Are there unnecessary noises from an open window?

- Is there enough room?

The environment is critical, especially when applying physical intervention, especially in cases where individuals may not be willing to have such intervention applied.

This chapter has demonstrated a good level of required knowledge surrounding limitations and accountabilities when supporting individuals exhibiting challenging behaviour. We now recognise the importance of staff training, the importance of using the least restrictive option, and the importance of risk assessments.

RECORDING AND REPORTING INCIDENTS OF CHALLENGING BEHAVIOUR:

It is important to record and report incidents of behaviour that is challenging. In any responsible environment of care, it is important to record and report incidents. That is why in any hospital or general practice, the first point of call will always be to record the name of the person coming in. To record is to write or set in a manner that what is written can be referred by others later, or it can be something that can be used as reported. There are various ways of recording or record-keeping: writing, taping, videoing.

1). THERE ARE METHODS OF RECORDING CHALLENGING BEHAVIOUR INCIDENTS:

Through this study we learn that the use of the ABC chart is most commonly used. First developed for schools, the ABC abbreviation is known as:

(A) ANTECEDENT;

Refers to triggers, anxiety signals, and distress that may have happened to the individual as a start or cause; the immediate occurrence prior to the challenging behaviour.

(B) BEHAVIOUR;

A succinct, definitive, and exact description of the challenging behaviour as how and when it takes place.

(C) CONSEQUENCES;

This is about the aftermath of the challenging behaviour that occurred; it records any concluding factors, why the challenging behaviour took place, and how it was dealt with.

The ABC therefore will be a chart including the relevant information:

- Date and time

- Name of individual

- Behaviour

- Consequences

- Interpretation of behaviour

- Strategies applied and strategies to prevent recurrence of negative behaviour

How to use an ABC chart in the childcare setting:

In childcare we use the ABC chart as an observational tool allowing us to record information about a particular behaviour:

- In our childcare setting the aim of using an ABC chart, also known as the tracker, is to better understand what communication the behaviour is making from each child and report on that child accurately.

- Therefore in the acronym ABC, the 'A' refers to the antecedent or the event that occurred before the behaviour started. We record what the child was doing, which carer was in charge, who else was there, where the carer and the other people were; we record any sights/sounds/smells/temperatures/number of people that were present or in the vicinity and the environment and also what their proximity was.

- In the acronym 'B' refers to an objective way and clear description of the behaviour that took place or occurred, e.g. Child John threw a book against a wall.

- In the acronym 'C' refers to what occurred following or after the behaviour or the consequence of the behaviour, e.g. the other children moved away from Child John, sightings of people or objects present, noise levels in the room increased or decreased.

In childcare guidance shows that it is important to decide on one or two target behaviours to record initially. The childminder or teacher placing the ABC chart in an accessible place to make it easier to use after the target behaviour has been resolved.

When the teacher has finished recording the behaviour on several dates or numerous occasions is when to check for triggers or situations where the behaviour is most likely to occur using the evidence on the chart:

- When/what time has the behaviour been most likely occurring?

- What happens or during what activities is the behaviour most likely taking place?

- Evidence of any times or activities during which the behaviour does not take place

- Whereabouts or in what room is the behaviour most likely to happen?

- With which people, e.g. teachers or other children, is the behaviour most likely to take place?

- It is very important to examine and record what consequences might be sustaining or exacerbating the behaviour:

- It is important to highlight what the behaviour achieves for the child, why they do what they do.

- We examine if the child avoids or escapes from any learning activity by engaging in the behaviour.

- We examine if the child is rewarded in any way by engaging in the behaviour.

- We examine what the child is attempting to communicate to carers/teachers by engaging in this behaviour.

When the SENCO, childminder, or teacher has identified the triggers for the behaviour and the consequences that may be upholding or maintaining the behaviour we are now ready to develop a behaviour support plan: by using the ABC chart we consider:

i). Any alternative or more appropriate skill we can teach the child in order to take away by elimination their need to engage in this behaviour

ii). Any changes that we can introduce or make to the environment or the child's timetable (schedule) so that we decrease the child's exposure to the trigger

iii). Reflecting, have we addressed the need that the child was trying to communicate?

iv). We examine the appropriateness of any need for a reward/incentive scheme in the short term.

v). In childcare, we have to ensure that we have communicated the plan to everyone who will be caring for the child.

2. THERE IS ALSO THE STAR APPROACH WHICH IS AN ACRONYM FOR:

- Settings; in the setting carers observe the individuals and the behaviour; also take account of environment.

- Triggers; the carers look out for triggers, monitor and work to minimise or reduce likelihood of triggers of challenging behaviour.

- Actions; the carers take appropriate actions to manage behaviour and support individuals towards full potential.

- Results; the carers will observe the results of interventions.

For best practice, recording using the STAR process enables the carer to record accurately when (time), where (setting), and the what (incident) and report on it accurately.

The STAR approach of recording and reporting will incorporate the following information:

1. Defines the occurrence and the behaviour

2. What achievement or result takes place from the behaviour?

3. What the triggers or causes are of the behaviour

4. What the environment is like wherein the behaviour takes place

5. What personal causes/triggers precipitate the behaviour?

6. What contributes to the occurrence of the behaviour, such as skills deficiencies with the carer or the individual?

The carer using the STAR approach can then highlight strengths and weaknesses, identifying not just skills deficits but also areas for the individual to get more support.

Therefore, it is important to record and report incidents of behaviour that is challenging.

RISK ASSESSMENT:

Reporting on incidents helps with risk assessment: the incidents are recorded therefore there is a point of reference and lessons are learned: through this course we learn that "risk assessment is the process of evaluation of the potential consequences that may be involved in any projected activity".

When risk assessment is being done:

1. Consideration of specific personal factors:

- Medical conditions of the individual with challenging behaviour

- Physical or mental disabilities

- Emotional or sensory issues

2. Consideration of environmental factors:

- Lighting

- Heating or cold/temperatures

- Noise or other distractions

3. Consideration of situation factors:

- Proximity of other people in the room

- Will anyone interact with the individual?

4. Consideration of background factors:

- Is there a history of when and how the behaviour starts?

- If there had been issues of self-harming, attempting it, or threatening it

- If there had been threats or issues of harming other people

- If the individuals self-neglect

- If the behaviour can exacerbate or escalate rapidly

5. Consideration of high-risk factors:

- If the individual is suicidal

Whilst observing and recording to report incidents, it must be noted if the behaviour was contained, and whilst the individual may have been restricted (if so), it was at a minimum. The dignity, liberty, was taken into account and balanced with the safety of the individual and others.

Therefore, it is important to record and report incidents of behaviour that is challenging; considering the reports help with risk assessments and support planning. As part of reporting incidents in childcare we have to inform parents of any accidents or incidents however minor and this is done in writing: it has to be done in an effective way:

Effective reporting of incidents and injuries entails the use of:

- The incident or accident log/book

- The recording in a diary of when and what happened and informing colleagues

- The accident/incident forms such as ones designed in the childcare setting (children refer to these as bump notes) which they take home to inform the parent

The incident: if resulting in injuries, the law requires through the Health and Safety Executive to report the following:

- If injury causes loss of sight

- If injury is a result of a crush

- If injury has been the result of burns

- If injury is scalping and causes attendance at hospital

- If injury caused unconsciousness resulting from asphyxia or injury to the head

Therefore, it is important to record and report incidents of behaviour that is challenging; considering the reports help with risk assessments and support planning.

CHAPTER 13

The challenge to recognise the benefits of reflection following episodes of challenging behaviour

REFLECTION ON AN INCIDENT CAN ASSIST IN MANAGING FUTURE BEHAVIOUR

Reflection on an incident can assist in managing future behaviour: this is the result of having learned lessons from experience or the past. Carers share effective strategies that have been previously used. Past incidents help carers to deal more effectively with incidents in the future. Interventions are applied more appropriately in view of their past effectiveness. A carer must be an effective and competent reflector.

What reflection does for the carer includes the following points:

Helps to inform planning and actions

Helps carers look back, rectify mistakes, learn lessons, and improve practice

Helps carers to develop current and future roles

Helps improve confidence and practice

The cyclical reflection process is defined as cyclic as to winds round and repeats same actions in reflection:

The cyclical reflection process enables the carer not just to reflect but ponder and plan for the incidences, how and when they occurred, and what plan for the best practice of the future. The cyclical process includes the following elements of reflective action:

- The description of incidents, what took place, happened, or occurred

- The feelings of those involved, what was thought, heard, or tasted

- The evaluation of the issue, whether it was positive or negative, contradictory or constructive

- The analysis of the incident/event, whether it made any sense or what sense, meaning, is made out of the incident

- The conclusion of the event/incident and scoping for any further action

- The action planning wherein we put forward strategies and outcomes prospective for the future, next time

Through this study we understand the use of reflective practices: the study details the "Gary Rolfe et al." model of reflective actions: the model works through three areas of practice, namely:

1. The model asks the question "what" in addressing the problem or issues of challenging behaviour.

- What the problem is

- What role or part did I take or play in the situation?

- What achievement was I trying to make?

- What were my actions or inactions?

- What response did others make in the situation?

- What were the outcomes or consequences for all people in the situation?

- What thoughts, feelings, emotions did the incident give rise to?

- What were the positive and negative or good and bad experiences?

2. The "Gary Rolfe et al." model of reflective practice then leads into the "so what question" or in the words "where do I fit in?".

The parent or carer has had the impression of what the problem is, so what:

- So what information does this experience give me, teach me, or how does it inform my practice?

- So what were the bases of the things I did, my actions?

- So what else do I know that I can make bear on the circumstances?

- So what would I have done differently to make the situation better?

- So what is my current information and comprehension of the situation, with new information?

- So what is the wider picture, what issues, and any new developments in the circumstances?

3. The "Gary Rolfe et al." model of reflective practice then leads into the "now what question" or in the words "what can I fit in?".

The parent or carer has had the impression of what the problem is, now what:

- What does the parent or carer have to do now to ensure that the behaviour improves or the situation is made better?

- What considerations do I have to make now for the bigger picture or new developments to make this action a success?

- What are the likely consequences now from the actions I have taken?

In applying the what factor to the situation, we learn how reflection on an incident can assist in managing future behaviour. The study guides us through various aspects and components that make reflection necessary for the carer in practice with individuals of challenging behaviour:

The necessity of reflection helps carers:

- To uphold standards at a high level

- To maintain the quality of service

- To work in a way reflecting the legislation for care

- To maintain strategies and actions within the care policies

- To self-examine and grow in the work ethic, development of the practice

- To work well with others and positively aim to achieve set goals

The necessity of reflection will identify areas of personal carer development which will then be met by:

1. Parent or/and care worker training courses

2. The carer liaising with colleagues and their managers/supervisors

3. Using the internet appropriately

4. Using books, periodicals, and care journals

5. By referencing with the official guidance and legislation

Reflective practice enables service users, care workers, and the patients/individuals to contribute thoughts and share impressions which allow the care to be improved and standards to be held high. This is how reflection on incidents can assist in managing future behaviour. This enables carers to identify aspects of development, the areas where more or new learning can be done in the provision of care.

Identifying development areas:

A carer's reflective practice enriches the skills the carer employs and harnesses in work. The reflective methods help inform the practice; the attitude and knowledge acquired enables good and strong analyses of how well the carer performed in particular areas of care. Those carers, the patients, and others involved in the issues of challenging behaviour:

- To comprehend their own intentions, values and aspirations

- To emotionally prepare when faced with challenging behaviour and any distresses

- To handle and manage sudden or unexpected incidents

- To manage any potentially moral conundrums and unexpected situations

- To inject innovative thought when faced with new situations

- To notice when any things are not right, not working well, and act swiftly with confidence to arrest the situation

- To be best at comprehending any limits as a carer

With these aspects in motion, therefore, reflection on an incident can assist in managing future behaviour: this is the result of having learned lessons from experience or the past. Carers share effective strategies that have been previously used. Past incidents help carers to deal more effectively with incidents in the future.

The challenge of how you would describe your own reactions to challenging behaviour

Care brings about emotional reactions. In my childcare situation; own emotional reaction to behaviour that challenges for instance caring for a child who has difficulty adapting to changes of just joining the pre-school class, handling frustrations, and problem solving; may initially draw sympathy which grows into empathy and then valuing the child with care. Emotions building into constructive care makes the carer get to the point of what happens next, as that child learns to solve problems together with his parents and teacher. The carer's human reaction may come naturally, but the carer's practice and any carer's emotional skills will be important in a situation of challenging behaviour.

The emotional feelings may include the following:

a). Feeling guilty where the carer may acknowledge that they did not do enough or take sufficient intervention. This study suggests that where carers respond to accidents the guilty emotion will occur.

b). Anguish is that reaction when the carer gets verbally abused or deliberately angered; taunts and insults cause carers to become angry. Many times in childcare a parent refuses to comply with policies, e.g. of timekeeping, and when attempts are made to discuss the situation, why the parent does not collect the child on time, that parent could become abusive, not taking into account that carers too have children and a life outside the job of care.

c). Feeling fearful is a normal reaction to circumstances of threats: challenging behaviour is apparently threatening and carers can become fearful due to physical attacks or threats.

d). Shocking emotions are a result of the threatening experience especially when the behaviour is sudden and takes the carer by surprise, emanating from an individual that is normally or usually calm, something out of character. Therefore the carer must always expect the unexpected where there is challenging behaviour.

e). Relief: Carers can be relieved, and relief emotions can occur even just by changing a work shift, if the shift has been so volatile. Relief is classed as the strongest emotion in human beings.

f). Failure; where carers have been in a situation of challenging behaviour and all strategies applied do not work, it is possible for carers to feel that they have failed, yet the carer has the next step of referral to better equipped professionals. But that referral may not take away the dejection of the failure emotion.

g). Disbelief; this is a state of emotion that combines surprise and horror. A carer feels emotionally horrified for instance in cases where the individual with behaviour that challenges begins to be violent, threatening to harm others as well as self-harm.

h). Satisfaction; to support a client from behaviour that challenges, to a state where the behaviour becomes positive, is something to celebrate; the carer will feel emotionally satisfied. Appropriate training and work or practice experience enables the carer to manage the supports appropriate to dealing with any of the emotions that arise in the case of management of challenging behaviour.

To deal with emotions demands self-awareness, so that the carer is aware they are or are becoming emotional in order to manage their own emotions.

The parent or carer's awareness of their own limitations:

The parent and carer must understand and know their own parental and carer position through self-awareness.

The carers must consider their own experience and exposure to incidents of challenging behaviour.

The parent or carer through self-awareness must ask, what limitations do I have and do my limitations prevent me to care competently?

The parent or carer can control emotions, but must ask, "Am I frightened of the volatile nature of behaviour?"

The parent or carer can control emotions by being self-aware, asking, "Am I trained, and therefore skilled to do this work?"

The parent or carer through self-awareness and reflection is able to self-assert that; "I am prepared and I am controlling my own emotions. I am supporting the individual who has volatile behaviour."

Self-awareness, awareness, and reflection enables the parent, or carer, to call for support or use referral to others in order to avoid doing what they (carer) are not trained or equipped for. Carers using reflection and self-awareness prevent harm or injury to self or others as they (carers) know what they can and cannot do. Therefore a carer should always control emotions and not act emotionally whilst helping to support individuals who exhibit behaviour that challenges.

Non-emotional involvement:

The carer draws from reflection and self-awareness that the role is supreme, the role of a carer, being here to support behaviour, to enable individuals to full potential. A carer therefore using skills learned and drawing from work experience should always practice controlling emotions and not act emotionally whilst helping to support individuals who exhibit behaviour that challenges: the "importance of being non-emotionally involved" is that the carer can work in spite of the volatile state of affairs caused by challenging behaviour from the client:

- The client may use abusive and racist or discriminative language directed at the carer, yet the carer has not got to emotionally react to the abuses, but carry on the work, and use the strategies of support and call in colleagues where the carer feels threatened.

- The individual/client may use swearing directed at the carer, yet the carer has not got to emotionally react to the swearing, but carry on the work, and use the strategies of support and call in colleagues where the carer feels threatened.

- The client may use offensive posturing such as spitting at the carer yet the carer has not got to emotionally react to the spitting, but carry on the work, and use the strategies of support and call in colleagues where the carer feels threatened.

- The client/individual may use self-harm, cutting oneself, yet the carer has not got to emotionally react to the self-harm, but carry on the work to manage the behaviour, and use the strategies of support and call in colleagues who have the skills to administer interventions that can subdue the individual from the volatility of self-harm.

- The client may use abusive and discriminative language, taunting a carer who may have a disability, yet the carer using skills of self-awareness and reflection has not got to emotionally react to the abuses, but carry on the work, and use the strategies of support and call in colleagues where the carer feels threatened.

This book teaches you that parents and carers should not act instinctively, but professionally and skilfully: anger should not overtake a parent or carer; a parent or carer must not abandon the child or client/individual because if a parent or carer abandons an individual with challenging behaviour, the individual is at risk, the act of abandonment demeans that individual, the individual is disrespected and loses dignity. Therefore the importance of being non-emotionally involved is part of a carer's own skill and forms part of the carer's professional reactions to behaviour that challenges.

The carer should seek support after an incident:

Debriefing is part of professional conduct: in some incidents that cause strong emotional reactions to carers, where the carer feels s/he cannot cope or the incident provokes much emotional feeling, it makes sense to seek support and counselling to come to terms with that experience:

The situations that are likely to evoke such extreme distressing emotional reactions may include:

Extreme road accident injuries

Fatalities of extreme casualties from motorway accidents

House fires with extreme burns and injuries to inhabitants

Drowning casualties

Landslide or avalanche casualties

Terror attacks in cities

These extreme situations cause distress and provoke strong reactions to those who witness them; carers such as ambulance responders may be among the first witnesses. It is thereafter that a carer may have feelings of distress and trauma which necessitate debriefing and talking through their experience to cope with such a memory: there are individuals that can be points of contact for carers to seek support including:

1. The carer can seek support from "family members of a friend".

2. The carer can seek support from "supervisor or line-manager".

3. The carer can seek support from "doctor or a GP".

4. The carer can seek support from "a professional counsellor".

5. The carer can seek support from "a colleague".

6. The carer can seek support from" a representative of the union".

The carer can seek support from "any of the above" and where appropriate professional support where appropriate techniques for management of emotions and reactions to extreme distressing incidents can be dealt with.

CHAPTER 14

There is a challenge of consequences of your own actions when involved in incidents of challenging behaviour

CONSEQUENCES OF OWN CONDUCT:

<u>The consequences of your own actions when involved in incidents of challenging behaviour:</u>

We learn that any action by a carer when dealing with challenging behaviour will incur consequences.

Desired consequences of a carer's actions ensure that there is no poor response to the behaviour:

- Positive behaviour is the desired effect of any support from carers.

- Maintaining the dignity of an individual is the desired effect of any support from carers.

- A calm quality of life is the desired effect of any support from carers.

- Ultimately, the recovery to full potential is the desired effect of any support from carers.

The desired effect or consequence is the result of the carer's cored, skilful, and professional actions taken with reflection and self-awareness.

Actions of a carer must be wrapped in self-awareness and reflective skill which comes from being:

- Equipped with appropriate training

- Ability to manage own emotional feelings

When the carer is able to manage their own emotional feeling, the consequences would be management of the situation of challenging behaviour and ensuring it does not escalate. Therefore, the consequences of poor or undesirable responses by a carer to challenging behaviour give rise for all involved to be at risk.

<u>Effects of poor response:</u>

Where the parent or carers do not self-reflect and do not use self-awareness of who they are, what their role is, it may result into behavioural escalation due to:

- The carer disrespecting the individual maybe by reacting emotionally to abuse from the client

- The carer may unskilfully make the individual feel loss of self-esteem or dignity

Carer training therefore imposes that the carers must be cognisant of the following:

- Never react or respond emotionally to volatile actions from a client.

- Never retaliate to verbal or physical challenges of a client. The carer must be self-aware of legal and professional consequences.

- Never engage in a slanging match or argument. The carer needs to know that the individual is someone distressed and any more stress can escalate the behaviour that challenges.

- Never laugh at an individual with challenging behaviour; it is disrespectful to laugh at people. If the laughter makes the individual angry, the challenging behaviour would escalate.

- Never shout at the client; it is not respectful or dignified if shouted at. Many individuals with challenging behaviour can find shouting intimidating and frightening and this causes escalation of behaviour.

- Never walk away as a carer's task is to support the individual, not walking away from them. Walking away is defined as breaching the duty of care.

- Never cause the situation to escalate by any action or reaction. As a carer use:

+ Avoidance skills to ensure the situation does not escalate

+ Avoid disrespecting the individual who has challenging behaviour

+ Avoid becoming emotionally involved or losing the self-awareness and reflective skills

+ Avoid anything, any reaction, that can cause escalation of the behaviour

Where if necessary the carer finds they are unable to cope they must call for or seek assistance from colleagues or the multi-agency support.

<u>When a carer should seek assistance and support:</u>

Self-awareness makes the carer professionally reflective, knowing that as a carer, there is a duty to care. A carer cannot walk away, but seek assistance if the volatility of behaviour is such that the carer cannot deal alone.

- Is the situation getting out of my control?

- The effective recognition of self-awareness is assessment and analysis of the situation and if a situation is one the carer cannot deal with then strategies to call in assistance.

- Carers can have code words to respond to various situations, and such a word can be broadcast on an intercom or the pressing of an emergency button will generate response and required assistance in an establishment of care.

- In care, to seek assistance is strength not failure or weakness.

- To seek assistance demonstrates self-awareness and reflective professionalism.

Therefore a parent or carer who is not going to breach the duty of care knows and understands when to seek assistance. Where carers seek support and assistance it reduces the likelihood of self-harm or injury to individuals with behaviour that challenges, and those that care for them.

Reducing risk:

Self-awareness is important to reduce risk to oneself as a parent or carer, but also reduces the likelihood of increasing the causes of escalating the behaviour and this study teaches us with examples of the risks that could be avoided, e.g.

- The individual could physically self-harm or injure other people.

- The individual with challenging behaviour or others could be emotionally harmed.

- The individual could be subjected to loss of respect and dignity by the carer's lack of self-awareness.

- The individual with challenging behaviour could be the subject of physical intervention unjustifiably or illegally if the carer is not self-aware and reflective.

- The individual could be unnecessarily distressed if the carer was not self-aware.

This book suggests further that action taken against a carer could be put in place by the individual who is being cared for; this could be an official complaint against the carer. Therefore the things the carers do should be only those that reduce but don't intensify risk to self, the individual/client, or others.

The challenge of supporting individuals to understand their behaviour in terms of the following:

Reviewing what occurred directly with the individual is how to support individuals to understand their behaviour in terms of events and feelings leading up to it:

- Carers must ask the individual how that individual felt before the incident.

- Carers must ask the individual if that individual felt distressed.

- Carers must ask the individual if that individual was feeling frustrated prior to the incident.

- Carers must ask the individual whether s/he was feeling anxiety.

- Carers must ask the individual if anyone else was with them.

Through this debriefing exercise the carers will ascertain what the trigger was. This is partly how to support individuals to understand their behaviour in terms of events and feelings leading to it.

b) Their actions

Reviewing the individual's actions contributes to how to support individuals to understand their behaviour in terms of their actions: the carer to effectively review the individual's actions must:

- Give sufficient time for the individual to go through the debriefing process

- Ascertain if the individual will effectively communicate, what language or communication method the individual prefers

- Then help the individual to explain what the individual was doing when the incident developed

- Establish how the incident developed through a question and answer process

- Allow for the individual to say as much as they wish to

- Ascertain how the individual felt at the time of the incident

- Allow time, so that nothing negative is left bottled up

- Ensure that no negative feelings are expressed and nothing is likely to trigger the incident again during this process

c) The consequences of their behaviour

Knowing the consequences of the individual's behaviour is how to support individuals to understand their behaviour in terms of the consequences of behaviour: the carer has a duty to explain things to the individual so that:

- The individual knows that there are consequences for behaviour.

- The individual is not punished for the occurrences of the incident.

- The individual is not rewarded for negative behaviours.

- The carer must be harnessing consequences suited for each individual.

CHAPTER 15

The challenge of the range of support services available to those involved in episodes of challenging behaviour

THE RANGE OF SUPPORT SERVICES

It is yet another challenge for a parent or a carer to muster the range of support services available. The range of support services available to those involved in episodes of behaviour that is challenging is an important aspect of ensuring the welfare of carers and other frontline staff that respond to challenging behaviour: the role of carer can cause anxiety and stress. Stress and anxiety resulting from the nature of experiences that carers have to deal with make it necessary that there are a range of support services, to help the carers and others that work in such situations when they cannot cope with particular issues that they have had to deal with in the duty of care. The range of support services available to those involved in episodes of behaviour that is challenging can be some or a combination of the following:

1. Carers can use "effective debriefing" which is:

+ Usually part of their normal scheduled supervision

+ Set up purposely after an event or incident that is particularly acute

+ Set up to help the carer to identify areas of development or personal training

+ Set up to reassure the carer and build their confidence

The carer may have identified their own deficiency in an area of care; they share this information with their supervisor or manager.

2. Colleague-to-colleague support; this is also part of the range of support services available to those involved in episodes of behaviour that is challenging;

+ Good working relations are critical to ensure that staff support one another.

+ Sharing information can be very reassuring.

+ Staff get to understand that they are not the only ones who have faced a traumatic or bad incident.

+ Staff get to know that others too get affected by what they see.

+ Staff get to understand that the role is challenging everyone involved.

3. Carer mentoring and supervision; during supervision it is important that:

+ The carer and the supervisor work with honesty

+ Deal with weaknesses and strengths in a sincere manner, with constructive criticism

+ Pick up any issues and signs where the carer may not be coping well

+ Examine how the role is affecting the carer

+ If needed the carer can ask for and/or be referred or signposted, e.g. for counselling

4. Staff appraisals: regular staff appraisal will strengthen the carers in their role. Appraisals help:

+ Dialogue regarding the role of the carer

+ Discuss potential for upskilling or development

+ Identify what aspects of the skills needed may be lacking

+ Carers to openly and frankly discuss their role and map out positive steps forward

5. Upskill and keeping up to date with career training: the carer needs boosting of skills in order to:

+ Be confident as s/he delivers care

+ Be reassured as they evaluate and self-assess how well they are doing in the role

+ Increase in self-esteem

+ Make achievement through knowledge and extension of skills horizons

+ Avoid suffering role-related stress

6. Holding a meeting with a union representative; to discuss issues with a union representative will:

+ Assist the carer to bounce ideas on how to proceed on matters relating to the role of the carer

+ Help clarify the role and the matters that could or might cause stress

+ Allow the union to intervene with objectivity; e.g. to ensure the employer allocates work within the confines of the job description

+ Also, if appropriate, make signposting

Therefore there are numerous support mechanisms that can be used by care workers in cases where they have difficulty coping with their role.

Significance of monitoring good practice:

To monitor the "good practice" is important.

To monitor good practice is what enables care workers to share ideas.

To monitor good practice is what enables staff to become more effective in care roles using the ideas they share.

To monitor good practice is what enables enhancement of quality of life for clients/individuals they care for.

To monitor good practice is what enables carers to gain confidence.

To monitor good practice is what enables and upholds the policies and procedures of care.

To monitor good practice is what enables and encourages a carer's positive attitude.

To monitor good practice is what enables reduction of frustration in the workforce.

To monitor good practice is what enables the sharing of methods of good practice.

What enables to monitor good practice is the result of formal and informal meetings through debriefing is how the carers share information may be done in how they respond or react to specified incidents, either through informal chats between colleagues or formal meetings.

The monitoring of good practice is what enables things or actions, care that improves the quality of life, through application of care, by care workers; helping to support positive behaviour of individuals who have challenging behaviour.

There is therefore a range of support services available to those involved in episodes of behaviour that is challenging. This is an important aspect of ensuring the welfare of carers and other frontline staff that respond to challenging behaviour.

There is support from other professionals:

There is support from other professionals wherein the range of support services are available to those involved in episodes of behaviour that is challenging, which makes it an important aspect of ensuring the welfare of carers and other frontline staff that respond to challenging behaviour:

(A) The doctor (GP): is the primary point of contact when a carer feels ill.

- The illness could be physical or mental.

- Diagnosis is made of what is causing illness for the carer.

- GP may make referral to another service, for instance a counsellor.

- Medication may be prescribed.

(B) The counsellor: provides a non-judgemental and empathetic environment.

- Carers can discuss the issues causing stress.

- Counsellors do not order carers or patients on what to do.

- Counsellors will empower carers in analysing their own situations and making their own decisions.

- Counsellors help the carers make decisions on how to proceed in light of the situation.

- Counsellors help the carer build stamina and their own resilience and would know what measures to take should the situation reoccur.

(C) The other form of therapists:

There are options when sought by carers who experience stress. This study suggests that a (CBT) cognitive-behavioural therapist may be one such option to enable carers to deal with, manage, and overcome the stress.

(D) Supported self-help groups:

A self-help group is one usually set up by people who identify with others who experience similar incidents. Many cities or localities have stress-related self-help groups in the UK, and this brings people together to share experiences of what triggers their stress, but also enables them to share ideas of managing and dealing with stress. Such self-help can reduce stress.

There is the above listed support from other professionals as well as self-help wherein the range of support services are available to those involved in episodes of behaviour that is challenging, which makes it an important aspect of ensuring the welfare of carers and other frontline staff that respond to challenging behaviour.

The challenge of support systems available to maintain own well-being.

The support systems available to maintain own well-being will support the carer in such a way that:

- A carer would maintain and seek out supports for their own well-being.

- Well-being is a state of being healthy, happy, and comfortable.

- When a carer uses the systems available to support own well-being, this brings about satisfaction.

- The carer must understand and have the knowledge that stress can be overwhelming and stress makes it difficult to maintain well-being; therefore a carer must always seek out the ways, the support systems, available to maintain well-being.

It is important that in order to maintain well-being the carer or any person alive should:

+ Be participating in society, making connections, and therefore socially active

+ Be using their bodily functions to full potential; such that they are physically active

+ Be using one's awareness of present, future, and the past but not becoming overly focussed and stressed by any

+ Be free with openness towards new experiences, learning lessons of life, celebrating life

+ Be sharing and living life through kindness and giving with other human beings

The moment the carer or any person is not fully enjoying the above elements of life they should seek support in order to maintain that well-being.

PATTERNS OF THE SYSTEMS OF SUPPORT:

Stress takes away productivity and positive attitude from a carer, however the carer can draw from the following support system:

1. Techniques of self-help: It is the carer using self-found methods for the reduction of distress or stress. Many find discovery of new things to do, writing, going to the gym, going to self-help groups of similar people, developing and writing down in a diary or inventory of experiences in order to share them. Self-help is the most significant of the systems available as everything almost depends on the sufferer/carer to make the first move, seeking or responding to offers of help.

2. Techniques of relaxing: the carer when experiencing symptoms of stress can take up things like breathing exercises, yoga, or a game, taking up things that help the carer to relax; these may for some be slow walks in a park or swimming.

3. Dialogue or speaking to other people: The carer can seek out other people who have had or still have similar circumstances in order to overcome the isolation associated with stress. Through talking with others reassurance is gained by both. Through this many people find the necessary signposting they may not have been aware of.

4. Self-reflection: The carer must be self-aware, conscious of one's well-being and when to take action, to discuss the matter with others. Self-reflection will enable a carer to know what triggers the stress. Once the source of stress, be it work related or forces external from work, is identified, then the carer can identify with others the potential strategies that can help manage and cope with stress.

Therefore the above are good examples of the support systems available to maintain own well-being which will support the parent or any carer.

STRATEGIES OF COPING WITH STRESS:

Working with individuals that have challenging behaviour causes stress for carers; carers must be able to cope with stress:

+ Coping strategies enable the carer to best cope or manage their anxiety, and overall stress.

+ Coping strategies will reduce emotional reactions when a carer is working in a demanding environment.

+ Coping strategies enable the carer to terminate the progress of the stress.

This book suggests the following examples of coping strategies that can form part of the support systems available to maintain own well-being which will support the carer:

A). Knowledge and expertise sharing:

+ Carers who share knowledge and expertise have raised self-esteem.

+ Carers who share knowledge and expertise find themselves valued and appreciated.

+ Carers who are appreciated want to repeat what they are appreciated for.

+ Carers when valued will feel good.

+ Appreciation is a reward.

Therefore the carer sharing knowledge and expertise with others and who is appreciated is using that strategy to cope well within the role of a carer. This is evident usually when parents with children that have, e.g. ADHD meet and share their experiences on how they deal with particular issues with their children. The parent is the most suitable carer since the parent knows that child better than anyone else could.

B). Solid networks of support:

+ Carers can have a friend, someone or anyone else with whom to share the difficulty.

+ Carers draw emotional satisfaction and strength by sharing, e.g. with a partner or colleague what is happening at work.

+ Carers who have a positive relation will benefit from a solid network of support.

Therefore the carer using solid networks, sharing knowledge and expertise with others, and who is appreciated is using that strategy to cope well within the role of a carer.

C). Managing expectations and setting realistic goals:

+ Carers must learn to set targets that are not too high in order not to fail achieving them.

+ Carers must learn not to put too much undue pressure on themselves.

+ Carers must learn not to become inadequate resulting from taking on too much which cannot be done or would not be done well.

+ Carers must avoid stressfulness from over-exertion.

+ Carers will do well to discuss expectations, challenges, and goals in order to manage them realistically.

Therefore the carer managing expectations and setting realistic goals will be sharing knowledge and expertise with others and is appreciated and is using that strategy to cope well within the role of a carer.

D). Recognition of fear and other limitations:

+ Self-awareness of what apprehensions a carer has is important in order to have training on the matter.

+ Limitations of dislikes and likes is critical for a carer, in order to have training on the matter.

+ Anything that would make the carer unable to play their role of carer to full potential should be recognised in order to have training on the matter.

Therefore the parent or carer by recognising fears and limitations will be managing expectations and setting realistic goals which will be sharing knowledge and expertise with others and is appreciated. The carer would be using that strategy to cope well within the role of a carer.

The challenge to know the importance of accessing appropriate support systems.

Pass this challenge or meet this challenge head on and you will excel as a parent or carer.

The importance of accessing appropriate support systems is significant in parenting and care work.

To clarify or explain the importance of accessing appropriate support systems for stress-related issues in a parent's or carer's life is best started with defining what stress is:

What is stress then?

= Stress is simply when the parent or carer or any person cannot cope with the conditions of circumstances that are.

.

= Stress is when a parent, carer, or person's ability to deal with circumstances is different from what they perceive to be the circumstances.

= Stress is when the parent, carer, or person feels that their ability to respond to a situation is stretched beyond their ability.

Workplace Stress:

For the carer, causes of workplace stress will include the following:

- Expectations and targets or goals set unrealistically, for instance where there is no resource or equipment to use to meet the need.

- If managerial support is lacking, the carer at the frontline may not know how to proceed in a situation.

- When the carer feels inadequate and unprofessional, this makes the carer incompetent and will stress any worker at all levels.

- If carers are not appreciated for good work, ignored for promotion, and never consulted, this can make them lose motivation.

- Extra and unrealistic workload; such extra demands would cause stress as the carer juggles time and work.

- If carers are not trained or prepared for a task and yet made to do it, it stresses them.

- When activities are beyond the control of a parent or a carer, this lack of control causes stress.

- If there is any bullying or harassment in the workplace against a carer, it will cause stress.

- When the overall working environment is poor, carers will become stressed.

Parental Stress:

Parents stress as a result of various responsibilities. Some of the responsibilities demand that a parent takes care of multiple siblings. It is hard to deal with a child who has challenging behaviour. It is not easy to keep multiple appointments for the children given the multiplicity of specialists that deal with the many conditions surrounding challenging behaviour.

A parent's workplace is not only at home, but also covers all the other places where the child goes to get various services. The parental work is 24-7. We must therefore know that very many parents with children who have challenging behaviour do not have enough sleep or rest, have less financial resources as they cannot economically participate due to the overbearing demands of care. The parent often neglects their own welfare, not wilfully, but due to overwhelming demands. Therefore the parent must maximise the available multiple agencies and engage with them. The parent must deal with the child with love, but as a professional care work in order that s/he can manage stress.

Therefore in the care for children or individuals with behaviour that challenges, it is important for the carer to deal with their own welfare, well-being, to ensure that they as a carer can access appropriate support systems to enable them to manage the stress so that it does not escalate. Therefore the signs and symptoms of stress should well be identified and addressed.

Symptoms and signs of stress:

= High blood pressure

= Increased heart rate

= Breathing problems

= Aches and pains

= Problems of indigestion

= Insomnia; the problems of sleeping, the lack of it and excess of it

= Feeling nauseated frequently

= Problems of diarrhoea and/or constipation

= Feelings of fatigue, constantly

= Uncontrollable losses or gains of weight

Controlling and monitoring oneself for the above symptoms of stress will help a carer; as it is important for the carer to deal with their own welfare and well-being to ensure that they as a carer can access appropriate support systems to enable them to manage the stress so that it does not escalate. Therefore the signs and symptoms of stress should well be identified and addressed. Alongside the above mentioned signs and symptoms there are psychological and emotional symptoms and signs that announce the onset of stress in a carer when working with individuals with challenging behaviour:

Psychological and emotional symptoms and signs that announce the onset of stress in a carer:

These will include the following:

~ Senility; loss of memory or general memory problems

~ Indecision: finding it to make options or decisions

~ Poor or lack of concentration

~ Being irritable, getting angry and upset at anything and everything

~ Worrying, overwhelmed, and feeling low

~ Developing a state of wariness and frustration

~ Insecurity, unnecessary feelings of suspiciousness of other people

~ Behaving in a manner that blows situations out of proportion; overreacting

~ Beginning either to overeat or under-eating

~ Loss of appropriate motivation levels, feeling lethargic, and not wanting to do or act at all

For appropriate controlling and monitoring oneself for the above psychological and emotional symptoms of stress, it will help a carer to know that it is important for the carer to deal with their own welfare and well-being to ensure that they as a carer can access appropriate support systems to enable them to manage the stress so that it does not escalate. Therefore the signs and symptoms of stress should well be identified and addressed. Alongside the above mentioned psychological and emotional symptoms and signs that announce the onset of stress in a carer when working with individuals with challenging behaviour, it is important to know what the consequences of stress are:

Consequences of stress:

The role of a carer for individuals with challenging behaviour has more demands. It is argued that some degree of stress actually motivates and enables the carer to be focussed on the job, but there are instances of stress which must be dealt with so that they do not impact negatively on the carer. This is a list of those areas of stress that can have negative impacts:

= When the carer begins to experience "increased susceptibility to physical illness" resulting from stress

= If the carer begins to feel "depression, anxiety and other mental illnesses" resulting from stressfulness

= When the carer starts feeling "reduction in job satisfaction" resulting from stressfulness

= If the carer feels "increased anticipation of accidents or putting clients at risk" resulting from stressfulness

= Where the carer feels there are "poor levels of communication" resulting from stressfulness

= If the carer develops "poor eating habits and lack of exercise" resulting from stressfulness

= When the carer begins to feel "isolation" resulting from stressfulness

The carer or any person being mindful of their own welfare:

- Should seek out the most effective methods of stress management

- Should seek out the avoidance of negative ways of coping with stress

In order for the carer to manage psychological and emotional symptoms and signs that announce the onset of stress in a carer when working with individuals with challenging behaviour, the carer should be mindful of their own welfare and know the importance of well-being.

Significance of well-being:

The significance of well-being is critical to doing or performing any responsible role in life: carers must use positive techniques to sustain their own well-being when caring for individuals who have challenging behaviour. There are a number of strategies that can be harnessed by the carer including:

1. **If the carer used "yoga and Pilates":** the combination can assist with physical fitness including the boosting of serotonin hormones and help in de-stressing.

2. **The carer can use "mindfulness":** This enables one to refrain from worry of or about unreal situations when they have not occurred. It also supports the individual to focus on the present, not what if, what could, or would be.

3. **The carer must** "connect with others" through building positive relationships, being a social individual, loving and accepting to be loved; this builds a network of friends with whom to share life's hardships and with whom to enjoy the joys of life; this enables management of stress.

4. **If from time to time a carer will ensure** "having a healthy lifestyle" checking and planning what they eat, when and how they eat, when and how they play or take physical exercise, being clean and healthy; the boost of health is through overall good feeling which is a result of bodily releases of good-feel hormones from exercise and enjoyment.

5. **Where a carer has "a hobby"** they find escape from the routine of work; hobbies become distraction factors from focussing on stress. It is argued that idling in thought about negativity can increase stress, yet a hobby can reduce stress.

6. Well-being can be enhanced by "me-time or taking time out" to do things trivial, play, or relax not tending to work, not worrying about work, but just enjoying life. This reduces stress.

7. The welfare of a carer can be increased by self-care, whilst also "helping other people"; doing some voluntary or community work in a local community centre can uplift spirits of others as well as one's own. For parents such can even be done with the child by going to enjoy places that the child likes.

8. The carer who is mindful of their own well-being will "be positive" in outlook; this helps personal focussing on positive occurrences in life, becoming more appreciative of the good and dealing with the bad when it happens. This way the individual will manage stress and reduce it.

9. The carer that takes time to "sleep well" allocating oneself ample or enough time for sleep will reduce stress by avoiding to stay up at night, long hours of work during day. Irritability and fatigue cause stress, and are results of restlessness. Sleep provides the best way to rest.

10. Ultimately a carer who is conscious of self-wellness will "recognise if help is needed and seek it" in moments of stress, and not allow the escalation of stress into mental illness:

- By identifying beginnings of stress the carer will draw from the support systems.

- By asking for help the carer will ensure sustenance of own wellness.

- By not ignoring even the slightest of stress symptoms but dealing with it, the carer ensures on welfare.

- By knowing that seeking help, guidance, or advice is good practice, and that experiencing stress is not a weakness or failure.

- By ensuring that stress is managed appropriately, the carer will sustain their own wellness.

It is therefore important to harness the support systems available to carers who care for individuals with behaviour that challenges.

The carer should avoid negativity in devising coping strategies:

This study shows the disparity of individuals who use positive and those that use negative strategies of coping with or managing stress:

When negative strategies are used by a carer, they abandon their own wellness:

- The carer will increase in stressfulness.

- The carer's stress will get worse.

- The carer's stress escalates and could be the basis for mental illness.

These negative strategies of coping with stress provide a false satisfaction and they include:

- The stress sufferer parent or carer starts drinking excessive amounts of caffeine.

- The stress sufferer parent or carer starts smoking, or even chain-smoking.

- The stress sufferer parent or carer begins drinking too much alcohol.

- The stress sufferer parent or carer develops gluttony and starts overeating or under-eating.

- The stress sufferer parent or carer starts compulsive spending of money, doing unnecessary shopping for instance.

- The stress sufferer parent or carer will feel unloved, unwanted, and isolate oneself.

- The stress sufferer parent or carer will be irritable and starts shouting at other people at the slightest of opportunities.

- The stress sufferer parent or carer could begin to self-harm.

- The stress sufferer parent or carer finds opportunity to be annoyed and argumentative, ready to fight, to harm others.

Depression and anxiety, obesity, serious physical illnesses, eating disorders can emerge from poor and negative strategies of stress management. Therefore a parent or carer who is self-aware, reflective, and understands the importance of wellness for self and others, should be able to seek help as appropriate to draw from a range of support opportunities for those who work with people who have challenging behaviour, in order to help those people and support them towards their full potential.

In conclusion it is extremely important for carers to access appropriate support systems when dealing with incidents of behaviour that challenges. This book has discussed the importance of having an appropriate support system to help relieve stress, anxiety, and to talk about how the parent or carer feels.

The book has also discussed the signs and symptoms of stress and what the consequences of stress are. This book has referred to "self-reflection" and "well-being" throughout and has made reference to the use of both positive and negative coping strategies and their effectiveness.

The information explained can be a daunting experience and can leave parents and carers feeling either of the two: empowered and positive; that they have supported and resolved a situation; or left feeling powerless and ineffective. However, one thing is clear, the book provides the necessary information for effective care and own well-being.

A colleague told me that her mother cared for the grandmother who suffered dementia for almost twenty years. The carer (a daughter) never asked for support (only got assistance from her husband). The carer felt that it was her duty to care for her mother and so never accepted any support from external agencies, friends, neighbours, or even family members. At times the carer who was a mother herself was worn out, angry (that no one in the family had stepped in), and emotional about seeing her mother deteriorate daily. She had the added pressure of also caring for her father who would reinforce to her that she was doing the right thing caring for his wife and that they "didn't need help". The colleague told me that she used to tell her mother that she and the dad needed extra support, they needed respite! Being offered help and accepting it is another matter. Over twenty years later, the carer mum wished she had accepted support and now knows the difficulties and emotions carers face.

In my childcare setting where I am a trustee, we have regular personal development meetings where we get to do the following exercises:

1. Analyse and reflect on what is required for competent, effective, and safe childcare practice, and provide active support for the team of employees.

2. Continually monitor, evaluate, and reflect on:

- Our knowledge and skills

- Our attitudes and behaviour

- Any experiences and personal beliefs that might affect our work

149

- How well we practice and what could be improved

- The processes and outcomes from our work

3. Seek constructive feedback to enable us to develop our practice, from:

- Parents, even the children and other individuals

- Key people

- Others that work with us or have contact within our childcare work

- Our supervisors

4. Identify any actions we need to take to develop and enhance our practice.

5. Identify the supervision and support systems available to us within or outside the organisation.

Recess and end notes

The challenge after getting a baby:

Many young people want to get a baby. No one teaches you or warns of the difficulties of having a baby.

No one tells you that baby may have a learning or developmental disability. Suddenly at the deep end after the baby is born, all sorts of things start to happen, the demand to feed, time to bath, nappy changes, illnesses, sleeplessness, juggling between childcare and work, stress sets in. A parent is instinctively, but also lessons learned from those who have done it before. Whatever the situation, a parent is the most qualified carer to look after their own child and all they need is resource and support from governments, experts in particular conditions.

Challenges of the usefulness of this book:

The usefulness of this book depends on the reader. My task as author has only been to pass on information learned through training and how it has been relevant to me: the book is how I have applied the lessons learned in my work. You will have found this book useful in whatever context or use you have read it. The challenges posed to society by challenging behaviour cannot be put in one book and summarised. These challenges will continue and the study of "challenging behaviour" is never ending. Let society open not only eyes and ears, but opinions and conclusions. One thing I have come to accept for sure is that for those who have challenging behaviour, they are trying to communicate something. But; can we see, are we listening to them, or are we preoccupied with opinions and conclusions of idealist scholars? Are we too quick to think there is a panacea, a tablet that can resolve the challenge which is ours as much as the individual suffers?

END NOTES:

The challenges live on and on and on…let us face them head on. My daughter that is autistic (nothing to be ashamed of) and aged eleven at the time responded to news of her auntie getting married in a very unique and different way from the rest of us: she felt she needed to interview the prospective husband before she could…let her auntie get married to him. (I would not have wished to be in his shoes…but the guy excelled): the following verbatim was the list of questions set for him:

30 Questions

1 Why did you chose to marry Auntie?

2 Why do you love her?

3 If you had to describe Auntie with one word what would it be?

4 Do you have a job?

5 How many gifts do you get her?

6 Is there going to be a cake at the wedding? (Mum said this question was really for me ☺☺☺)

7 What qualifications do you have?

8 Do you have a degree?

9 What does Auntie mean to you?

10 Are you willing to give her the best? Because Auntie is a princess in my country?!

11 Are you willing to follow my protocols?

12 Are you willing to make her happy and put a smile on her face every day?

13 If you are thinking of taking her somewhere you must let me know at all times?

14 What do you love about Auntie?

15 If you see another girl don't be naughty?

16 Will you always love her?

17 When did you propose to her?

18 How did you propose to her?

19 Do you have pride in anything?

20 After the wedding are you still going to treat her the same depending on how you feel for her?

22 After the wedding where are you planning to move?

23 Did you pass your GCSEs? If you didn't I'm going to have a word with you, Mister.

24 Did you go to university?

25 Do you have a driver's licence?

26 If you really love her will you take good care of her?

27 How do you know if Auntie loves you?

28 Do you promise never ever to hurt Auntie?

29 Did you pass your SATs?

30 Are you thinking of taking Auntie to a holiday after the wedding? Because I want to go too. Don't worry, I can fit into the adult suitcases easily or the other way round; Mister can go in the suitcase or I take his ticket. Don't worry, will buy ice cream sundaes, sit in a posh hotel…I can't wait.

If you say no, I'll do the puppy eyes.

Tip for men: bring a bouquet and lots of chocolates yum ☺☺☺

Whilst it was imposed on me to include this bit in the book, I have to acknowledge and thank my daughter, the author and interviewer; thank you for such a challenging and exceptional conclusion to this book.

CHALLENGES OF CHALLENGING BEHAVIOUR

However much you learn or get to know about challenging behaviour, there is always a new challenge to challenge your experience. The important lesson from this book is that "the carers" should look at the "sufferer with challenging behaviour" and ask themselves that; "what if I was the one in their place, how would I want to be dealt with?"